Psychological Trauma

Edited by Ana Starcevic

Published in London, United Kingdom

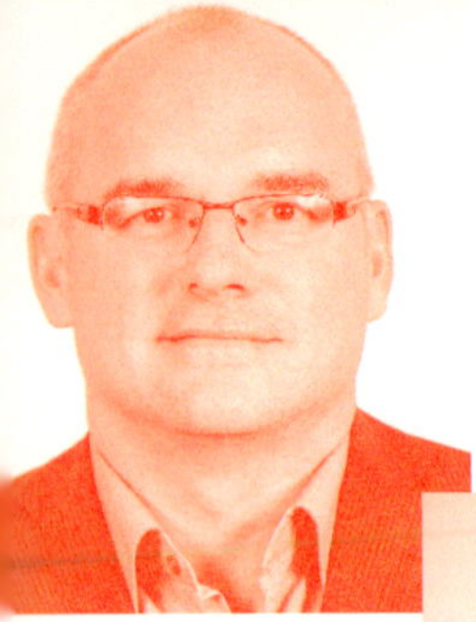
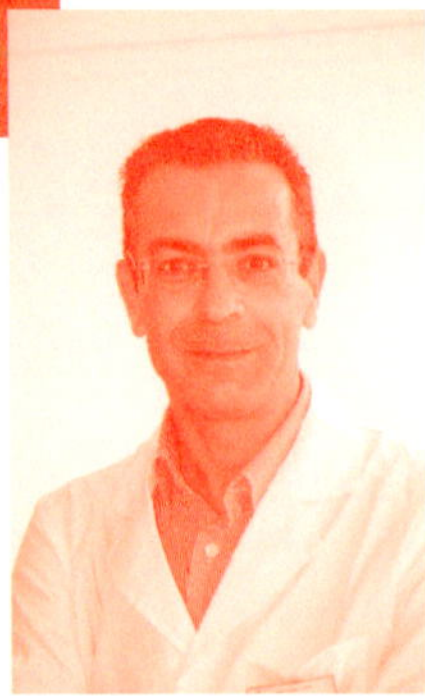
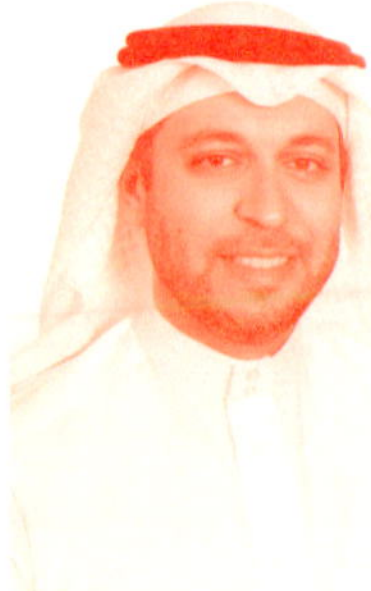
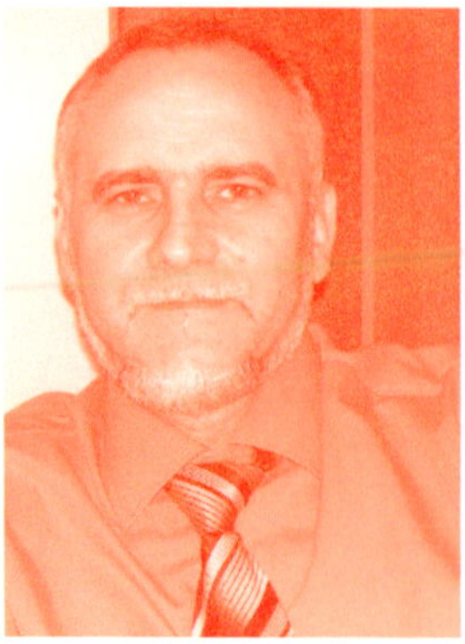
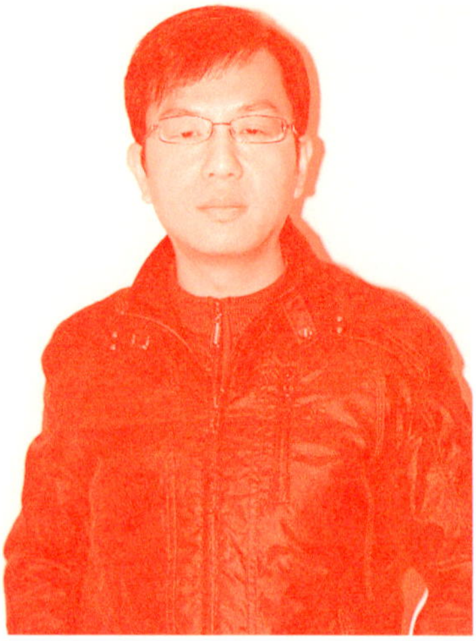
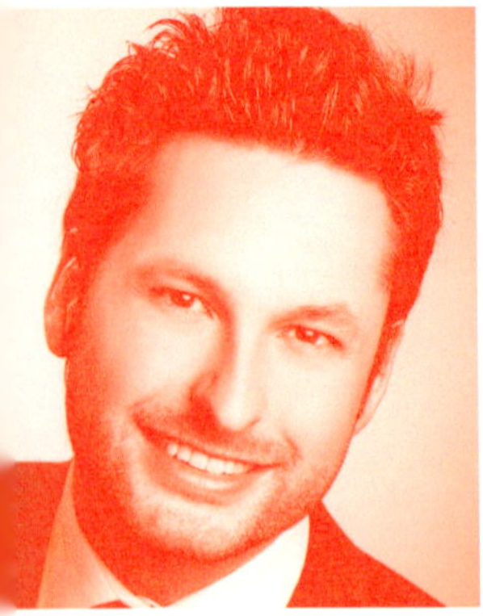
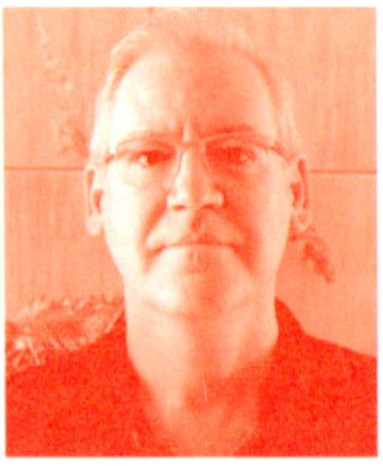

IntechOpen

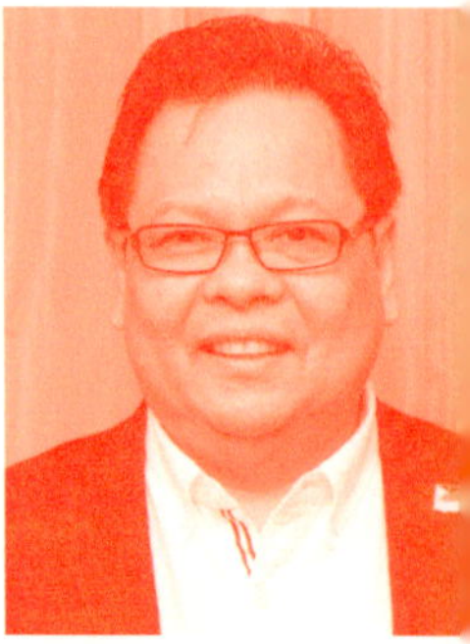
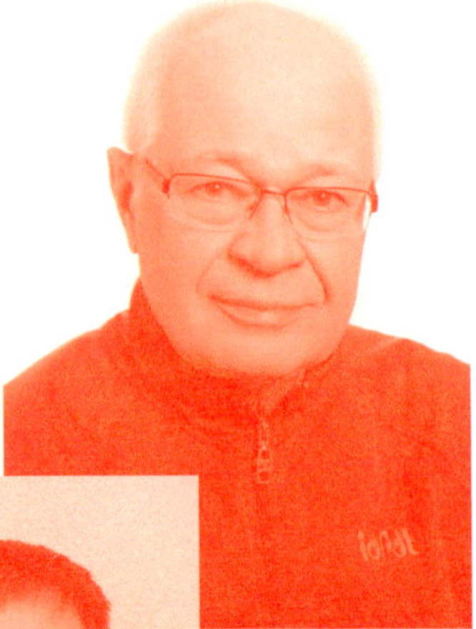
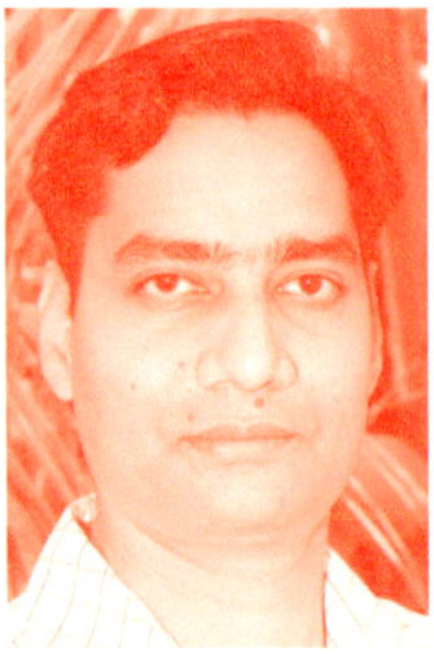
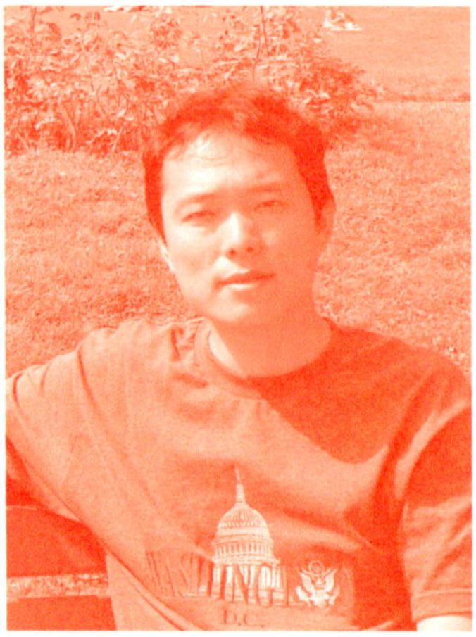
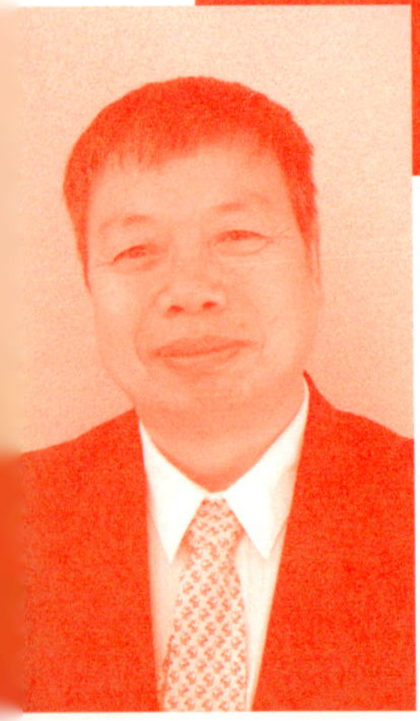
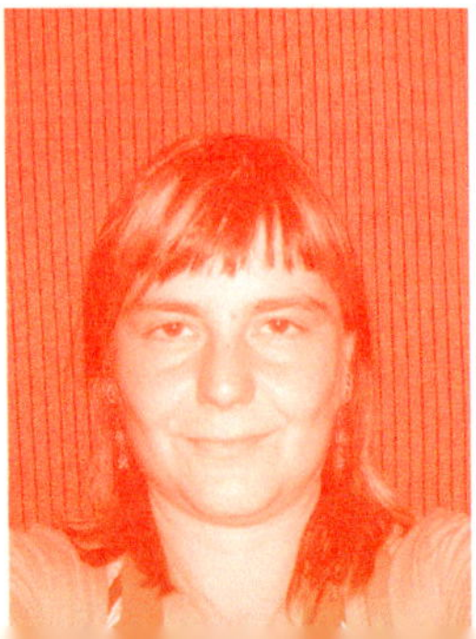

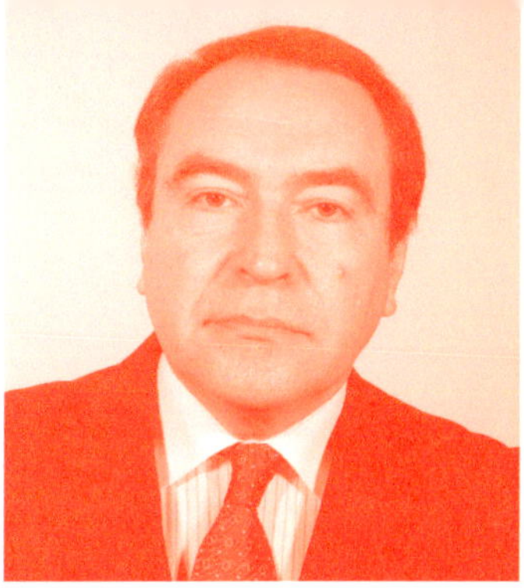

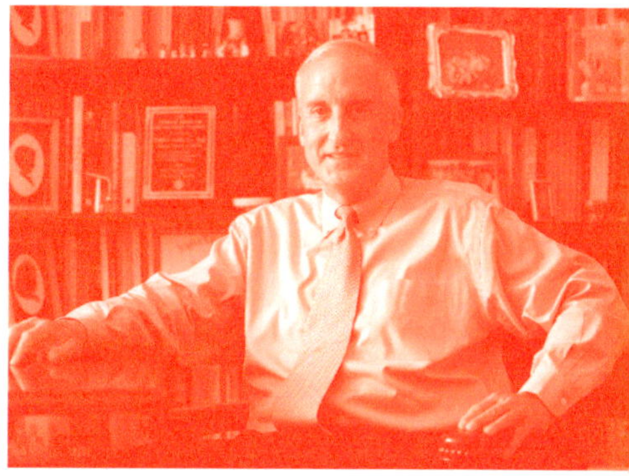

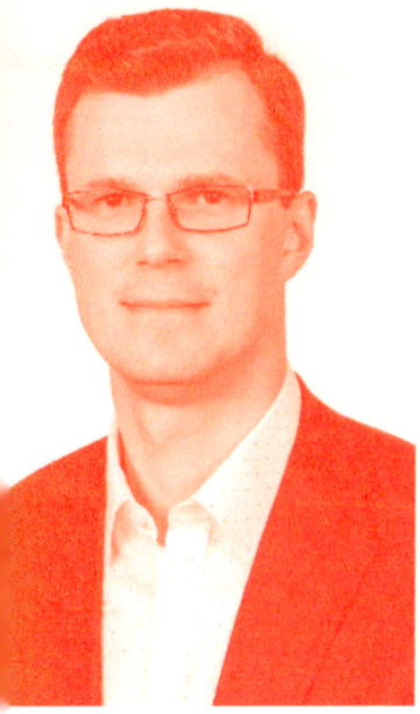

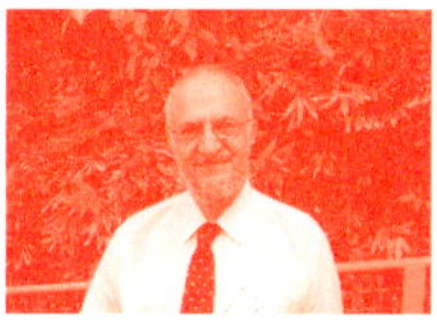

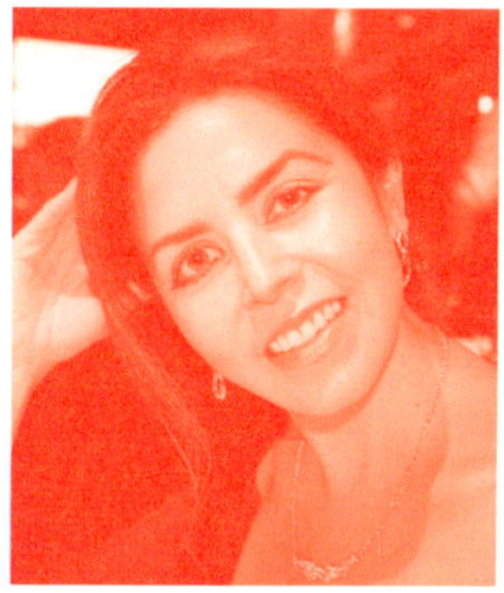

Supporting open minds since 2005

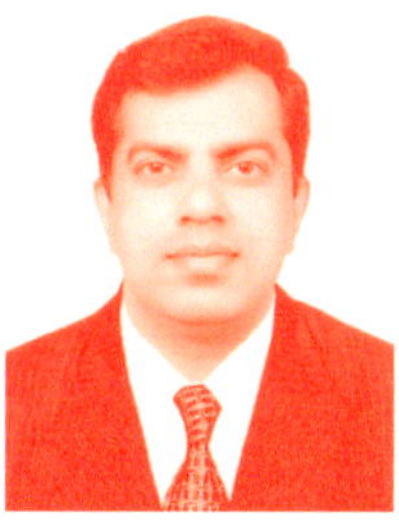

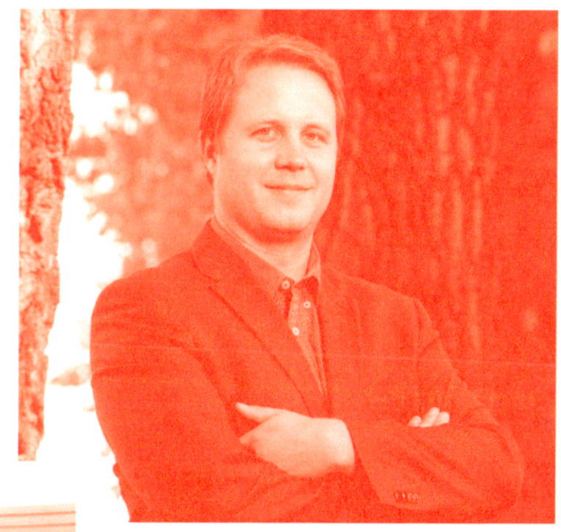

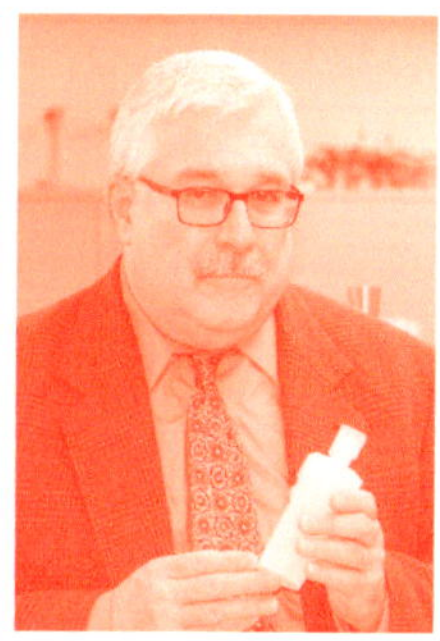

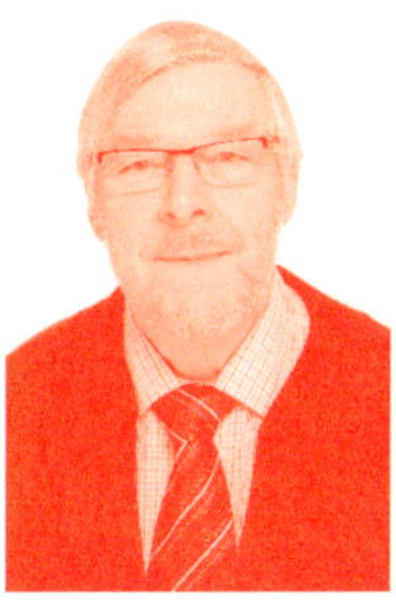

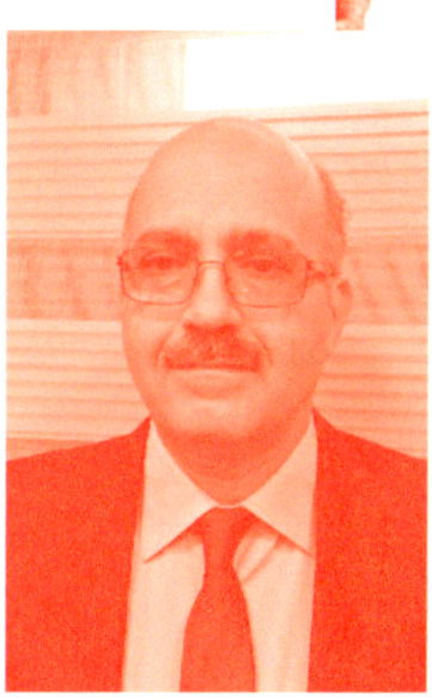

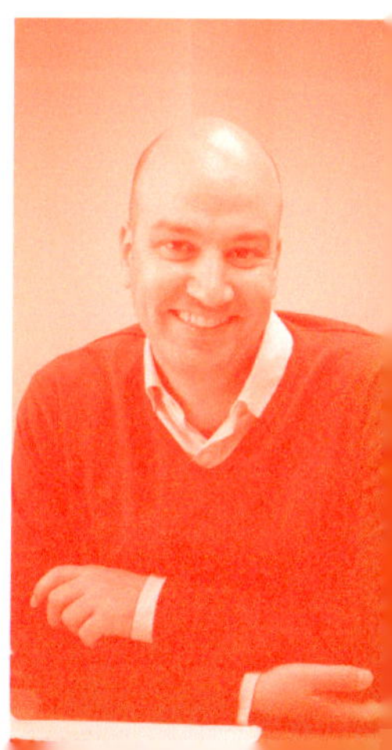

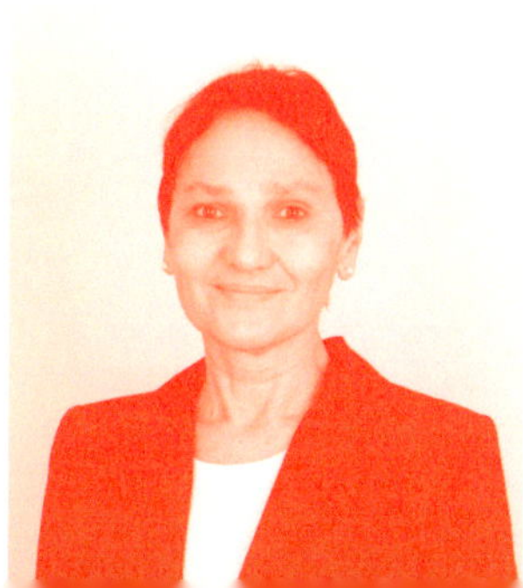

Psychological Trauma
http://dx.doi.org/10.5772/intechopen.77651
Edited by Ana Starcevic

Contributors
Catherine Athanasiadou-Lewis, Maria Uscinska, Andrea Polla Mattiot, Nicolo' Gagliano, Marion Trousselard, Célia Belrose, Lionel Gibert, Annemiek Van Dijke, Jacques Van Lankveld, Hiroshi Kunugi, Emiko Aizawa, Miho Ota, Ikki Ishida, Norie Koga, Shinji Sato, Takashi Asada, Kotaro Hattori, Shima Taheri, Maryam Ghasemi Sichani, Amirhosein Shabani, Ana Starcevic

First published in London, United Kingdom, 2019 by IntechOpen
IntechOpen is the global imprint of INTECHOPEN LIMITED, registered in England and Wales, registration number: 11086078, 7th floor, 10 Lower Thames Street, London, EC3R 6AF, United Kingdom
Printed in Croatia

British Library Cataloguing-in-Publication Data
A catalogue record for this book is available from the British Library

Additional hard and PDF copies can be obtained from orders@intechopen.com

Psychological Trauma
Edited by Ana Starcevic
p. cm.
Print ISBN 978-1-78984-369-9
Online ISBN 978-1-78984-370-5
eBook (PDF) ISBN 978-1-83962-804-7

For EU product safety concerns:
IN TECH d.o.o., Prolaz Marije Krucifikse Kozulić 3, 51000 Rijeka, Croatia,
info@intechopen.com or visit our website at intechopen.com.

Meet the editor

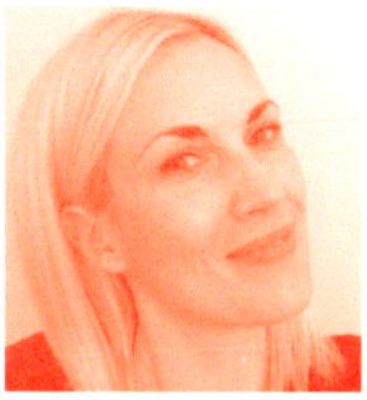

Dr. Ana Starcevic is an associate professor of anatomy and neuroanatomy, and a researcher at the Medical Faculty, University of Belgrade. She holds a PhD in Molecular Medicine and has extensive experience and expertise in basic and applied neuroscience. Neuroimaging was the main method of her PhD thesis, so her strong credentials in this area connect with the many scientific papers she has published in the area of brain morphology and its functions. She is the main author of two books and one chapter in the area of brain research; she has also authored a few neuroanatomical workbooks. She was a member of two projects investigating brain changes in different conditions. Dr. Starcevic is a psychiatry specialist who works with patients with different spectrum of stress disorders.

Contents

Preface

All emotions have physical effects but the ones that are suppressed under the surface are like ticking bombs, often called disorders in incubation. Individual trauma might result from a specific event or from a set of inconvenient situations that were experienced emotionally or physically, and are very harmful or threating to an individual. Some individuals have physical issues, some psychological, and some both. The term "trauma" originates from the Greek word trauma, which means wound. This term can be interpreted in the context of both physical and psychological wounding. Complex trauma presents an exposure to severe and repeated traumatic events or situations and also most often interpersonal nature. Emotional symptoms of trauma can vary, from shock and denial to irritability and mood swings. The persistence of shame, self-blame, sadness, and hopelessness can occur. Anxiety and fear are most often present when trauma happens. Except for the emotional, physical symptoms like insomnia or nightmares, fatigue, disturbed concentration, and muscle tension are manifested. Other symptoms include feeling suicidal, self-harm, and overreaction to even minor situations. Many studies have found that the more anxious and stressed people are, the more tense and constricted their muscles are, over time causing the muscles to become fatigued and inefficient. An abnormal reaction to an abnormal situation is a normal reaction. Trauma shifts brain network activity in many ways. Some brain structures involved in memory and cognitive functions are disturbed. Instead of being in good function, because of stress impact to the brain, default brain networks retune at rest and turn to unpleasantries. The negative cognitive bias we inherit, making threat detection a primary task, is amplified by unresolved trauma. The salient networks of the brain, which alter what we look for inside and outside, are disturbed and some of them are malfunctional. Emotional, physical trauma or both turn processing power away from working memory, making it harder for us to think clearly and emphasize the situational overreaction mode in an individual.

The impact of the influence of a traumatic event on an individual depends on the dynamics, duration, and severity of the specific trauma, as well as the subjective experience of the individual victim. One of the most important factors that plays a great role in shaping a person's perception and helps to respond to trauma situations is the past experience of the individual. It is the capacity to respond adequately and defend themselves. It is important to acknowledge that trauma does not only affect people directly involved during the exact time of its occurrence, but that its remnants could be carried over into the following generations.

In this book, the authors make an effort to present different perspectives of stress impact on the brain, its connectivity, and its consequences, which most often present as different psychiatric disorders and illnesses, most likely posttraumatic stress disorder and depression. Also, the authors present specific treatments for solving and resolving stress issues.

Knowledge of psychological trauma has been continually expanding in the literature and is applied in medical practice, but despite the establishment of a solid base of scientific literature on trauma and the growing modification of society and social media to the harmful psychological impact of traumatic events, this investigation area has yet to be incorporated in all areas of social awareness and life.

Ana Starcevic
University of Belgrade,
Serbia

Section 1

Introduction

Chapter 1

Introductory Chapter: Psychological Trauma

Ana Starcevic

1. Definition of trauma experience

Trauma generally presents a complex issue and we all know it all too well in its basic simplicity, but in other ways, we know nothing about trauma. Sometimes it can be heartbreaking and very difficult, but if we do not deal with trauma what is processing with us will keep going. Individual experience of a trauma event can be specifically related to different reactions of an individual to similar traumatic event and, of course, not all individuals who experience a potentially traumatic event will get psychologically traumatized. Most severe and nowadays very common for some individuals is to develop post-traumatic stress disorder after being experienced to some complex traumatic event. Coping mechanisms present maybe the most important parameter for an individual being traumatized to continue with normal life without any manifest or major consequences. Temperamental and environmental factors are the most influential from all the others.

Trauma is defined as an emotional response to an extremely negative situation. Trauma, as a physiological response to negative effects that impact the brain, can be so severe that they interfere person's ability to live a normal life, and help may be needed to treat the stress and caused by the trauma impact and to develop a person's state of emotional well-being.

2. Some of origins of psychological trauma

Traumatic experience creates psychological trauma when it overwhelms one's ability to cope with the situation and own emotions, and leaves that person fearing death, annihilation, mutilation, and the cause of traumatic experience most often include abuse of power, betrayal of trust, entrapment, helplessness, pain, confusion, and loss of something or someone very important in one's life. This consideration is very broad and it might include responds to specific violent events, accidents, and natural disasters, which are nowadays very common. Psychological trauma is also related to chronic and repetitive experiences, such as child abuse, neglect, combat, and constant deprivation. The term and situation that refers to it must be considered objectively, as it is up to each survivor to determine if it traumatic, as it can be manifested clinically by various psychiatric disorders. That means that two different individuals can experience the same provoke factor or situation which is mostly related as trauma, and one can be intensively traumatized and the other remain unscathed. It is really not possible to make one pattern or blanket generalizations. It can be different and highly specific from one individual to the next. Trauma comes in many forms, and there are differences among people who experience trauma, as not each brain is the same, its anatomy and physiology.

IntechOpen

3. Emotions

It is all about emotions. Emotions are very complex. Not only defined as one specific, maybe the most important mental function, based on discoveries made through neural mapping of highly specific limbic system structures, the neurobiological explanation of human emotion is that emotion is a pleasant or unpleasant mental state organized in the limbic system of the mammalian brain. Emotions are our feelings. Literally, we can feel the emotions as tingles, hot areas, and tension in different muscular region, especially posterior neck region. We must mention the cognitive aspects, but the physical sensation is what makes them really different.

They are described as a positive or negative influence that is commonly associated with a particular pattern of physiological activity and produce different physiological, behavioral, and cognitive changes that are often manifested in different brain structural changes as well as behavioral pathological patterns. Motivation of adaptive behavioral patterns would have contributed to its continuation in different ways, reproductive or psychological. Cognitive functions present very important aspects of emotion. Mental processes are still essential, particularly in the interpretation of events. Consciously experiencing an emotion is exhibiting a mental representation of that emotion from a past or hypothetical experience, which is linked back to a content state of pleasure or displeasure. The content states are established by verbal explanations of experiences, describing an internal state.

Emotions are complex. According to some theories, they are states of feeling that result in physical and psychological changes that influence our behavior. Emotions are closely linked to arousal of the central nervous system with different levels and strengths of arousal related to specific emotions and consequently to behavioral tendency. Like, extroverted people are more likely to be social and express their emotions; introverted people are more likely to be more socially withdrawn and settled in circle of their own emotions, often manifested as the driving force behind motivation. Controlling the emotions involve different components, such as subjective experience, cognitive processes, expressive behavior, psychophysiological changes, and instrumental behavior. The core of coping with psychological trauma is specific and appropriate identification of specific emotion and dealing with different components of emotion, as the most complex psychological function. In psychology and philosophy literature, emotion includes a subjective, conscious experience characterized primarily by psychophysiological expressions, biological reactions, and mental states.

Emotional and therefore psychological trauma is often manifested as the result of highly specific stressful life situations that shatter your sense of well-being, making you feel helpless in a dangerous world. Traumatic events often induce very strong feeling of life threat. Also, if any event makes an individual feel overwhelmed and isolated can result in trauma, and its psychophysiological aspects and clinical manifestations without any physical harm.

4. Effects on brain and its structures

All stress effects that can cause major pathological changes in brain physiology occur in different brain regions. The most affected is hippocampus and amygdala as well as prefrontal cortex and its interrupted connections with other brain areas and structures. It is not the objective circumstances that determine whether an event is traumatic, but your subjective emotional experience of the event. The more frightened and helpless you feel, the more likely you are to be traumatized. Trauma very often changes brain network activity and its patterns as default mode networks re-organizes activity mode of the brain as it drifts toward unpleasantries. It is considered that negative cognitive bias we inherit, making threat detection a primary task, is amplified by unresolved trauma, and brain networks are therefore prejudiced and compromised. Trauma draws processing brain energy in different directions from working memory, making it harder for us to think clearly. Sometimes, it is just like keeping the balance when talking about coping mechanisms and psychological trauma care. When evaluating and coping the psychological traumatic event, we must crucially consider loosing of dynamic balance of up to date dynamic connection between different brain regions that might be affected. Some are separated by dissociation, by an absence of connection, while others are over-connected, stuck together. Executive control networks are off-kilter [1].

Identification with trauma can be protective, but also make it hard to let go and move forward, which can be seen within the borderline personality disorder. Also, trauma can mimic narcissism, dependency, schizoid states, and so on, wearing many guises. In the situations when people fear to lose their identity, process of change is harder and it is not because we are about to lose ourselves, but because that is what we may fear and feel, the pain or re-experiencing the trauma event again, in our minds, which in summary present itself a symptom of trauma.

One of the best investigation results in the field of stress and trauma is the dose–response relationship which is related to one of the laws of physics, and that means the higher the dose of trauma experience is the more possible disturbing the consequences, which might lead to severe psychiatric stress-related disorders and illnesses [2, 3].

There are a lot of impacts that stress does to a human organisms, from beneficial to very critical and damaging. As at first it can be very stimulative, when increased and chronic, it can induce very serious changes in different brain structures, especially those involved in memory and cognition, which is most often manifested in different psychiatric disorders, such as PTSD and depression. Those brain structures are hippocampus, amygdala, prefrontal cortex, putamen, thalamus, and caudate nucleus, but as they are also interconnected with other brain structures, we cannot exclude other brain structures as they might be also involved [4, 5]. There are a lot of neuroimaging studies obtained, and these showed volumetric changes and defined neuroanatomical substrates in PTSD [6, 7].

5. Instead of conclusion

Therefore, a lot of research studies should be conducted in order to confirm, add, or decline the research results and findings till date. As we all learn new data from research studies about the stress impact and development of psychological trauma, we can add that they present synergy of biological, sociological, and genetic factors.

Author details

Ana Starcevic
Neuroanatomy, Medical Faculty, University of Belgrade, Belgrade, Serbia

*Address all correspondence to: ana.starcevic22@gmail.com

References

[1] Giller E. Passages to Prevention: Prevention across Life's Spectrum. 1999

[2] Nutt DJ, Malizia AL. Structural and functional brain changes in posttraumatic stress disorder. The Journal of Clinical Psychiatry. 2004;**65**(Suppl 1):11-17

[3] Rocha-Rego V, Pereira M, Oliveira L, Mendlowicz M, Fiszman A, Marques-Portella C, et al. Decreased premotor cortex volume in victims of urban violence with posttraumatic stress disorder. PLoS One. 2012;**7**(8):e42560. DOI: 10.1371/journal.pone.0042560

[4] Bremner JD. Traumatic stress: Effects on the brain. Dialogues in Clinical Neuroscience. 2006;**8**(4):445-461

[5] Bremner JD, Elzinga B, Schmahl C, Vermetten E. Structural and functional plasticity of the human brain in posttraumatic stress disorder. Progress in Brain Research. 2008;**167**:171-186

[6] Hull AM. Neuroimaging findings in post-traumatic stress disorder. Systematic review. The British Journal of Psychiatry: the Journal of Mental Science. 2002;**181**:102-110

[7] Koenigs M, Grafman J. Posttraumatic stress disorder: The role of medial prefrontal cortex and amygdala. The Neuroscientist. 2009;**15**(5):540-548. DOI: 10.1177/1073858409333072

Section 2

Psychological Trauma - Possible Causes and Underlying Pathological Mechanisms

Chapter 2

A Relational Perspective on Psychological Trauma: *The Ghost of the Unspent Love*

Catherine Athanasiadou-Lewis

Abstract

Psychological trauma is central to the practice of all psychological therapies and is possibly one of the most frequently uttered terms in the history of psychology since its philosophical inception by the Ancient Greeks. Despite the abundance of scholarship devoted to the study and conceptualization of trauma, it remains a perplexing phenomenon given that the majority of contemporary studies focus on post-traumatic symptomatology and allied diagnostic pathology. While the psychopathology of post-traumatic ramifications has been thoroughly examined, the pathopsychology of trauma remains an arena of ongoing exploration and debate. The purpose of the current chapter is to offer an overview of the most predominant conceptual frameworks of psychological trauma residing in the psychodynamic school of thought, which not only addresses the intrapsychic and interpersonal origins of traumatic pathology but also provides a normative framework of healthy human development. Alongside that, a clinical case vignette will be presented to illustrate the interventions, processes, and outcome of psychodynamic treatment for complex trauma. Positioned within a post-modernist paradigm, the chapter aims to review current psychodynamic literature from a perspective that supports the notion that reality can be interpreted in multiple ways and thus embraces the diversity of multiple analytical contributions to the study of trauma.

Keywords: psychological trauma, addictions, psychoanalysis, attachment, sexuality, love

1. Introduction

Derived from the Ancient Greek word 'trauma' (=wound) and preserved in its etymological originality, psychological trauma is a phenomenon that involves an injury to the psychological matter. *Trauma* is generally defined as any experience that is felt to be unbearable that shatters the human psychic potential and affects the human capacity to relate, and feel kinship with others authentically [1]. According to Kalsched, trauma refers to a type of psychological injury to the capacity to feel, which occurs when we are given more to experience than we can consciously bear, especially if we the lack resources to metabolise the mental states that emerge. Such an experience may disturb our sense of inhabiting the world in a coherent, safe, and meaningful manner [2]. As Greening quotes: *when we experience trauma, our relationship with existence itself is shattered* [3].

Traumatic experiences are broadly associated with a painful life event, which is characterised by its intensity, by the difficulty of the person to respond adequately to its sequalae and by its pathological long-lasting effects on the psychic organisation [4]. Thus, psychological trauma is the unique individual experience of a single event or enduring conditions, in which: (a) the individual's ability to integrate their affective experience is overwhelmed, and (b) the individual subjectively experiences a threat to life, psychosomatic integrity, or mental sanity [5]. The individual may be left feeling emotionally, cognitively, and physically overwhelmed, while common comorbid diagnoses associated with traumatic experiences include post-traumatic stress disorder, mood disorders, anxiety disorders, substance misuse, eating disorders and personality disorders.

The sequela of trauma commonly involves a sense of current threat, betrayal of trust, violation of psychological and somatic boundaries, loss of power, entrapment, helplessness, confusion, pain, dissociation and loss [5]. Broad examples of events that are associated with a traumatic sequela involve relatively impersonal events like natural disasters and accidents, or events of a personal character like many forms of abuse including psychological, sexual and physical assaults, wars and torture. Additionally, events of commission like interpersonal violation or events of omission like neglect and abandonment, which are not necessarily socially constructed as traumatic, may still result in the individual experiencing a sense of threat to their integrity.

The very fact that traumatisation is predominantly an esoteric, idiosyncratic experience renders notions of objectivity somewhat difficult to infer. For this reason, central to the formulation of traumatisation is an appreciation of the uniqueness of the individual's subjective lifeworld [6] and the conditions that may have been shattered as a result of exposure to psychologically wounding experiences. *It is the subjective experience of the objective events that constitutes the trauma...The more you believe you are endangered, the more traumatized you will be...Psychologically, the bottom line of trauma is overwhelming emotion and a feeling of utter helplessness. There may or may not be bodily injury, but psychological trauma is coupled with physiological upheaval that plays a leading role in the long-range effects* (Allen [6], p. 14).

At a neurobiological level, many studies have shown that the effects of environmental stress on the brain are being mediated through molecular and cellular mechanisms. Neuroimaging research findings found permanent structural changes in the prefrontal/frontal lobe volumes of the brain, as well as alterations in neurotransmitter systems in chronically maltreated children [7]. Additionally, rapid increase of dopamine under discrete or prolonged traumatic stress has been shown to cause DNA mutations in brain tissue. The main implication from these findings is that early repeated trauma may lead to permanent brain changes associated with psychopathology such as mood disorders. Even more crucially, Schore has highlighted the effects of relational trauma in the developing brain of the infant, by showing that early experiences of deprivation and neglect in the attachment system can result in an impairment of the limbic system and critical neuronal cell death, associated with future aggressive behaviour and affective dysregulation [8].

Over the years, a plethora of theoretical approaches and research studies examined the immediate and long-term psychosocial consequences of intensely traumatic events, and several psychological models have attempted to conceptualise and treat clinical presentations arising from traumatic experiences. Although psychotherapies began with traditional analytic approaches, other schools of therapy have examined post-traumatic syndromes like PTSD, including cognitive behavioural therapy (CBT), existential and humanistic counselling, dialectical behaviour therapy (DBT), and eye movement desensitisation and reprocessing (EMDR) therapy. Effective treatments for PTSD include trauma-focused cognitive-behavioural therapies, psychodynamic psychotherapy, existential-humanistic counselling, EMDR as well as integrative psychotherapies [9–14]. With the focus of the current chapter on psychological trauma rather than on PTSD, the ensuing discussion will address theoretical contributions from developmentally focussed approaches residing mainly in the psychoanalytic/ psychodynamic paradigm.

2. Historical overview of approaches to trauma

The relationship between trauma and mental illness was initially investigated by the French neurologist Jean Martin Charcot, who was treating traumatised women presenting with what was known as hysteria at the time (Greek *υστέρα* = uterus) in the Salpetriere hospital [14]. Hysteria referred to as a set of symptoms including amnesia, paralysis, convulsions and sensory loss that would be traditionally treated with hysterectomy. Charcot observed that these symptoms may have had a psychological origin and noted that traumatic events could induce a hypnotic state in his patients and was the first clinician who captured the process of post-traumatic dissociation owing to the endurance of unbearable experiences. Charcot's student, Pierre Janet, continued to examine the relationship between traumatic memories and dissociation. More specifically, Janet studied the impact of traumatic experiences on his patients' behaviour and personality development. Janet observed an association between his patients' intense affects and their recollections or interpretations of their traumatic experiences, and found that through hypnosis, abreaction and re-exposure to the traumatic memories, patients' symptoms were alleviated [14, 15]. A substantial contribution to the early studies of trauma arose from the works of Freud and Breuer cited in [16], starting with the famous case of Anna O, who initially presented with symptoms of hysteria but was later conceptualised as a case of dissociated, repressed trauma originating in her relationship with her father. In their studies on hysteria in 1893, Freud and Breuer referred to traumatic dissociation as *hypnoid hysteria* and highlighted its relationship to a traumatic antecedent. Implementing hypnotic techniques as an initial form of treatment led to the gradual development of the psychoanalytic approach with a focus on free association, abreaction and interpretation of unconscious intrapsychic and relational processes, as central to the treatment of traumatic presentations like hysteria [14]. In working with soldiers after World War I, Freud observed that his patients often re-enacted their battle experiences and noted that traumatic dreams have the characteristic of repeatedly bringing the patient back into the situation of his accident. In 1941, Kardiner, another psychoanalyst working with U.S. veterans from World War I, also studied the aftermath of trauma and his observations resembled Freud's and Ferenczi's postulations on the nature of *re-enactment*, a construct referring to an unconscious tendency to re-experience traumatic scripts: *the subject acts as if the original traumatic situation were still in existence and engages in protective devices which failed on the original occasion* (Kardiner [17], p. 82).

The enormous impact of the Vietnam War on the psychological well-being of soldiers inspired more organised studies on trauma [14], while a growing interest in traumatisation within civilian contexts, particularly abuse and domestic violence, eventually led to the development of a diagnostic classification of trauma-related syndromes known as post-traumatic stress disorder in the Diagnostic and Statistical Manual (DSM-III) [18].

2.1 PTSD vs. complex trauma

Post-traumatic stress disorder was originally classified as an anxiety disorder in the DSM-III and DSM-IV and is characterised by aversive experiences of anxiety, maladaptive behaviours, somatic symptoms as well as physiological responses that arise and develop following an individual's exposure to a psychologically traumatic event. Recent reviews in the diagnostic literature now classify PTSD within the trauma- and stressor-related disorders in the DSM-5. PTSD symptomatology as outlined in the diagnostic manuals is theorised to result in clinically significant distress or impairment in several aspects of life activity, like occupation, social relations and other major areas of everyday functioning [19].

Although the diagnosis of PTSD captures a set of symptoms related to post-traumatic syndromes, it does not address developmental causes and childhood antecedents, nor does it offer a more complex and comprehensive view of intrapsychic and psychosocial stressors that exert influence on personality development and trauma-related pathology or distress [14]. For this reason, trauma has been conceptualised as ontologically different to PTSD. According to McNally, naive realists posit PTSD as an objective, timeless, universal psychobiological entity emerging in response to extreme stressors, while social constructionists assert that it is a cultural artefact arising in the wake of the Vietnam War [20]. As Young quotes: *The disorder is not timeless, nor does it possess an intrinsic unity. Rather, it is glued together by the practices, technologies, and narratives with which it is diagnosed, studied, treated, and represented and by the various interests, institutions, and moral arguments that mobilized these efforts and resources* [21].

While trauma is always an antecedent to PTSD [20], the two are not synonymous and it is important to emphasise that PTSD does not capture post-traumatic manifestations in their entirety. While all PTSD sufferers will have experienced some form of injury at some point in their lives, not all traumatised individuals will go on to develop PTSD. Yehuda and McFarlane [22] have shown that psychological trauma does not necessarily lead to PTSD but may precipitate other symptoms and syndromes. The authors propose that factors not yet well understood determine the variability of individual responses to trauma. Numerous psychiatric diagnoses in addition to or other than PTSD have been identified in traumatised patients including depressive syndromes, anxiety disorders, dissociative disorders, borderline personality, and substance misuse [21]. Chertoff asserts that PTSD rarely occurs alone and suggests that a range of trauma-related psychological problems, not fully captured in the DSM-IV framework of PTSD, occur together, requiring a more comprehensive approach [23].

Responding to the epistemological limitations and challenges of PTSD syndromes, Herman [24] suggested that 'complex PTSD' should be included as a new diagnosis that would address the multiple origins of trauma and their impact on all aspects of a person's life including personality disorders. According to Herman, the lack of an accurate diagnostic concept has serious consequences for treatment, because the connection between the client's presenting symptoms and the traumatic experience is frequently lost. Attempts to fit patients into the mould of existing diagnostic constructs generally result, at best, in a partial understanding of the problem and a fragmented approach to treatment.

More recently, Ford and Courtois developed a more comprehensive model of 'complex trauma', conceptualising it as the *inability to self-regulate, self-organize, or draw upon relationships to regain self-integrity* (Ford and Courtois [25], p. 17). Complex trauma is *associated with histories of multiple traumatic stressors and exposure experiences, along with severe disturbances in primary caregiving relationships* (Ford and Courtois [25], p. 18). Therefore, a comprehensive formulation of complex trauma calls for a treatment model that addresses the immediate post-traumatic symptoms, which are not always limited or even relevant to PTSD but may instead manifest themselves in other clinical presentations. Additionally, the diversity of traumatic ramifications is fundamentally observed within the realm of human relationships and characterological formation. Because of the far-reaching implications of complex trauma for an individual, psychodynamic psychotherapy has been positioned in the literature as more effective for complicated types of PTSD and the broader interpersonal sequelae of trauma. Clinical and empirical evidence suggests that psychodynamic approaches may result in improved self-esteem, enhanced ability to resolve reactions to trauma through improved reflective functioning, increased reliance on mature defenses with concomitant decreased reliance on immature defenses, the internalization of more secure working models of relationships, and better social functioning [26].

3. Psychodynamic approaches to trauma

Much of the trauma literature in psychology has been based on classic psychoanalytic formulations [14], and later revisions include contemporary psychodynamic approaches, arising from the school of object-relations and interpersonal psychoanalysis [14–16]. In psychodynamic theory, trauma is understood to have a shuttering effect on the corporeality of the individual that requires psychological adaptation and results in a distinctive yet polymerous psychological sequelae. However, in comparison with competing theories, the psychodynamic model is distinctive in its emphasis on developmental history, unconscious function, and interpersonal processes [16].

Healthy human development throughout childhood is conditioned upon safe and stable interpersonal and contextual experiences, which shape the individual's intrapsychic dimensions and relational capacities. The interplay between the intrapsychic and the interpersonal determine to a large extent adult functioning and well-being, particularly in regards to one's sense of self and experience of the world around them [14]. Traumatic experiences hold the unique characteristic of interfering with children's natural developmental potential—that is, their ability to feel safe within their psychosomatic self and establish a sense of belonging within their human environment; to unequivocally experience mental states and authentically express them; to recognise others' mental states and empathically respond to them too; to imagine and to symbolise; to act autonomously but rely on others too; and finally to be able to love and create.

Freud's clinical observations led him to theorise that mental life is instinctually motivated by two oppositional drives—*Eros* and *Thanatos*. *Eros* literally translates into romantic love and *Thanatos* into death. For Freud, the interplay between the love instinct (also referred to as the life instinct) and the death instinct (aggression) is what produces intrapsychic conflict and results in anxiety and resultant pathology—*For it is through all bad feelings and conflicts are known* [27]. Freud chose his words with novelty. His reference to the life instinct as 'Eros' was not random as romantic love has been universally celebrated as the highest of all emotions. The idea that love is one of the most fundamental forces in the world, if not the most fundamental force, has a long and influential history [28]. Ancient Greek philosopher Empedocles argued that it was through love and strife that the four elements of nature—fire, water, air and earth—were bound together to create everything around us. Plato argued in the *Symposium* and the *Phaedrus* that love is our response to the forms—the higher form of reality, the model for everything that exists [28]. Plato defined love as *the joy of the good, the wonder of the wise and the amazement of*

Gods. But for Freud, the concept of love went far beyond affective experience—it necessitated an impelling function that preserved all the good for personality and civilization alike. For Plato, it is love that leads us to the forms, the ground of reality. For Freud, anything that we seek to understand and relate to, we invest with libido—in other words, we love [28]. Despite Freud's emphasis on the nature and function of the libido *per se* (the sexual drive and its symbolic expressions), he captured the importance of love both in intrapsychic and interpersonal terms predicating that love and reality are connected at the very deepest level [28].

3.1 Freud's theory on trauma

Freud's original *seduction theory* postulated actual sexual experiences during infancy and early childhood as the cause of all traumas and the basis for neurosis [16]. However, he lost faith in his 'seduction hypothesis' for a number of reasons: first, he came to doubt the prevalence of sexual abuse he encountered in his clinical practice, and second, during the course of his own self-analysis, his repressed sexual feelings towards his mother led him to acknowledge infantile sexuality as a driving force of personality development, from which he constructed the Oedipus complex. This revision led Freud to privilege the role of repressed unconscious fantasy and intrapsychic conflict over interpersonal factors in the development of traumatic neurosis [16]. Freud went on to distinguish between traumatic and anxiety neuroses on the basis of real occurrence versus unconscious fantasy and the resultant intrapsychic conflict (e.g., desire versus rage). According to Freud's clinical evaluations, the pathogenic agency was invested in the memory of the trauma and the patients' defences to tackle the emerging anxiety like denial, repression and dissociation. A discharged affect of the attached traumatic experience usually resulted in these memories transforming into tolerable ordinary recollections, accessible to the conscious mind. When a reaction discharge was, however, impossible, then these affectively undischarged memories were theorised to enter a *second consciousness* where they became secrets, either isolated from the conscious personality or available to it in a highly summarised form and often unconsciously acted out [29].

A related interpersonal observation was that of 'traumatic re-enactment'—the human tendency to repeat earlier patterns of relating in an attempt to master the conflict arising from the repressed, traumatic experience. Freud captured this phenomenon in his early writings on 'remembering, repeating and working through' [30] and termed it *compulsion to repeat* (Freud [30], p. 151). Attending to his patients' relational patterns using free association, Freud discovered the notion of transference, a relational phenomenon whereby the therapist (and other important people) symbolically represented a figure from the patient's past. By closely attending to the manifestations of the transference (e.g., how the patient treats the therapist, their expectations, wishes and anticipated roles) and gradually interpreting its aim (e.g., a wish to dominate an abusive parent by overpowering the therapist), Freud was the first clinician who attributed therapeutic change to the processes of the therapeutic relationship. *We must be prepared to find, therefore, that the patient yields to the compulsion to repeat, which now replaces the impulsion to remember, not only in his personal attitude to his doctor but also in every other activity and relationship, which may occupy his life at the time-if, for instance, he falls in love or undertakes a task or starts an enterprise during the treatment* (Freud [30], p. 151).

In addition to Freud's attendance to intrapsychic conflict and fantasy, the role of external traumatic experiences has been widely highlighted in the writings of many classical psychoanalysts including Carl Jung, Sandor Ferenczi, Anna Freud and Alfred Adler, all of whom emphasise the reality of early childhood traumatic experiences and their impact on the formation of mental representations of *self*

DOI: http://dx.doi.org/ 10.5772/intechopen.86375

and other. Followers of Freud like Klein, Winnicott, Fairnbairn and Bion developed his original model further and included the realm of human object relations, which is the centrality of relationships, particularly attachment processes and infancy experiences, in the formation of personality and character pathology following trauma.

3.2 Fairbairn's theory

A significant departure from Freud's conceptualisation of libido was offered by Ronald Fairbairn who believed that the libido was not *purely pleasure seeking* but *object seeking*, and as such, Eros could be understood as a drive for relational gratification [31]. When libidinal urges become thwarted in childhood, either via the frustration of the child's dependency strivings or because the child's efforts to establish affirming and safe interactions are not met in a reciprocal fashion by the care givers, the child turns away from external reality. *In place of those connections, the child creates a fantasy world of internal objects that contains features of the real-world objects with whom the child cannot establish and maintain a meaningful relationship* (Ringel and Blandell [14], p. 67).

Drawing on his work with abused children and schizoid presentations in adulthood, Fairbairn noted that traumatic experiences in infancy cause the developing child to feel unloved as a person in their own right and also to interpret their own love towards the caregivers as essentially bad, worthless or destructive. The child then absorbs the parental characteristics and identifies with the unresponsive features of the parents: isolated, depressed, masochistic, bullying and self-destructive [14]. Fairbairn asserted that by internalising these pathological character traits, the child re-establishes a connection to the parent, who is unavailable in other, healthier ways. *This type of internalization of the parents also necessarily creates a split in the ego: part of the self remains directed toward the real parents in the external world, seeking actual responses from them; part of the self is redirected toward the illusory parents as internal objects to which it is bound* (Mitchell and Black [31], p. 120) [14]. Traumatic re-enactments in subsequent relationships were thus associated with the painful sequelae of the object-seeking behaviour.

3.3 Ferenczi's contributions

Ferenczi's contributions to the theory of trauma equally favour experiences of exogenous nature and their exerting influence on personality development. Ferenczi studied phenomena of regression, repetition and acting out in treatment with abused patients, and apart from his emphasis on dynamics of the real traumatic relationship between the child and the perpetrator, he highlighted another important traumatic phase: the denial of the traumatic event by significant people in the child's life, most notably the child's mother. For Ferenczi, the environmental rejection of the child's living nightmare represented the most pathogenic component insofar as the child's reality was inadvertently invalidated, thus enhancing dissociation and depersonalisation leading the child to resort to distorting their own reality in order to survive. The problem with this type of defence is of course what Freud always referred to as the *return of the repressed* in the form of neurotic symptoms [14, 16, 32].

3.4 Winnicott's contributions

For Winnicott, the experience of trauma is central to the development of the 'false self', which comprises an inhibited, fragile and often hidden sense of identity, akin to an insecure attachment system, with an impoverished capacity for trust and authenticity [33]. In Winnicott words: *I find it useful to divide the world of people into two classes. There are those who were never 'let down' as babies and who are to that extent candidates for the enjoyment of life and of living. There are also those who did suffer traumatic experiences of the kind that result from environmental let down, and who must carry with them all their lives the memories of the state they were in at moments of disaster. These are candidates for lives of storm and stress and perhaps illness* (Winnicott [33], pp. 123–124).

Winnicott wrote that babies enter life with an 'inherited potential' for a 'true self' that reflects their existential essence [34]. In 'the holding environment' provided by an available, containing, responsive and emotionally attuned maternal figure, the baby's authentic, spontaneous expressions originating from the Id, develop and their sense of identity becomes firmly established. Infants, on the other hand, who are exposed to repeated deprivations or impingements, do survive but at the cost of 'living falsely'.

For Winnicott, the false self is a necessary facade that the child erects to secure the mother's love by being compliant with her inadequate adaptations or unconscious expectations. For example, a depressed mother might prematurely force an infant to be 'cheerful' and 'strong' by projecting all of her unconscious wishes for rescuing onto them; a child of very angry, unstable parents might be terrified from expressing any of its own darker emotions or a child of intrusive parents might be prevented from developing a capacity to be alone and regulate their emotions.

Winnicott's observations uniquely highlight the role of relational trauma in personality development, which is often subtle and invisible to 'the bare eye' as it does not necessarily encompass the drama of sexual or physical abuse and their visible scars, but instead runs within the psychic vein like a colourless poison.

3.5 Kohut's self-psychology

Kohut's self-psychology framework encompasses a novel model for understanding normative human development and developmental deviations, as well as a theory of psychopathology. At the centre of Kohut's theory is the idea that healthy personality development presupposes the satisfaction of core narcissistic needs within the attachment system, such as the need for mirroring (building a coherent sense of identity), idealisation (establishing self-esteem) and twinship (fostering a sense of belonging) [35]. Kohut viewed psychological disturbance as both originating and resulting in deficient self-functioning, manifesting in a variety of forms (e.g., borderline conditions, pathological narcissism and other personality disorders as well as depression, anxiety disorders and sexual perversions). Kohut formulated these conditions as the result of chronically occurring, traumatic breaches in parental bonds, most notably in empathic failures [14]. Unlike many object-relation theories in which maturity is equated with separation and individuation, self-psychology sees the developmental line of self-object relations as extending from birth to death [14]. Thus, self-psychology is predominantly an interpersonal approach that addresses intrapsychic development on the basis of how core narcissistic needs are being met within the attachment system.

3.6 Bowlby's attachment theory

The origins of attachment theory are found in Bowlby's idea that the relationship of close proximity between the infant and the primary caregiver serves not only as a survival mechanism, but it also allows the infant to develop socially and emotionally. In other words, the close proximity to protective caregivers keeps the child safe during threatening times, while psychologically it creates a sense of 'secure base', allowing the child to explore the environment. Influenced by object relations, Bowlby developed the concept of internal working models (IWM) to describe the representational models of self and others stemming from the quality of early bonding experiences. Traumatic attachments characterised by experiences of abandonment, physical or sexual abuse, neglect or parental indifference are theorised to hinder various domains of psychosocial development, such as romantic and peer relationships, disturb affect regulation, and damage the self-concept [14, 16]. Contemporary psychoanalysts, Fonagy and Target, introduced the term 'mentalisation' to describe one's ability to comprehend mental states in self and others (e.g., thoughts, feelings, intentions, and wishes) and developed a model that linked insufficient mentalising capacity to a pathological self-originating, in traumatic attachment, experiences [36].

4. Clinical vignette 'Olivia: *the ghost of the unspent love'*

This section will present a case study summarising elements of psychodynamic treatment, process and outcome with a particularly challenging clinical presentation of substance misuse following developmental trauma. To preserve confidentiality but to maintain originality of the essence of treatment, all identifying details have been replaced with fictitious information. I borrowed my title from a novel written by Maro Vamvounaki in 2008 *The phantom of the unspent love*, which uniquely highlights the intricacies of inner deprivation and psychic unfulfilment, in an era where satisfaction is pursued at all costs. As the novelist highlights: *Love is indeed the great completion of the existence, but only when it's about the love that you give.*

4.1 Olivia

Olivia was a 48-year-old consultant cardiologist who sought therapy following years of opiate dependency syndrome and episodes of recurrent depression. Olivia's distinguishing talent and formidable skill led her to a nomination to specialise as a heart surgeon, but due to her concealed heroin addiction, she 'settled' with cardiology alone (mainly teaching coupled with part-time consulting), acknowledging the potential risk involved were she to perform open heart surgeries. Olivia developed an addiction to smoking heroin (but never injecting) during her medical training and saw it as a way of forming peer relations and getting a sense of belonging when she was studying. Prior to smoking heroin, as a child, Olivia used to enjoy inhaling white spirit and reported doing so since the age of 9, when she started attending painting classes and spirit was largely available for art purposes. Her bizarre inhalant addiction went unnoticed by her immediate environment, and in the same fashion, Olivia kept her ongoing heroin abuse hidden, by controlling withdrawal symptoms before they would kick in. Olivia took substantial, intermittent breaks from her substance misuse that allowed her to maintain a reasonable level of professional and social functioning, but she eventually relapsed into her original habits, getting stuck into the vicious cycle of withdrawal and submission into cravings.

Olivia described a 'normal' childhood with plenty of material goods and toys, albeit dominated by parental conflict and fought relations within her family. She had some fond recollections of her mother as an affectionate and emotionally attuned figure but also described her as highly critical and controlling, often intruding into Olivia's space leaving her feeling anxious and hypervigilant. Her father, on the other hand, was described as a remote and somewhat mysterious figure, whose main interest was his business and professional success. Her father was also described as the main source of stability in the home, and Olivia admired him for his physical appearance, wealth, moral values, and for offering them a comfortable, middle-class upbringing. Olivia had very little recollections from her childhood overall and the father in particular, as after the age of 9, he started travelling abroad a lot and so his presence was not felt in their home but was not missed either.

Her mother portrayed the father as cold and indifferent and frequently accused him of cheating on her (without evidence), causing her to feel neglected and chronically depressed. Olivia would often console her mother's depression by keeping her entertained and by minimising the impact of her own neediness on her, by withdrawing or presenting content, despite feeling otherwise. Both parents held high aspirations from Olivia, and they hoped that she would study engineering in order to take over the family business in land development. While Olivia complied with their wishes and strived to please them, she chose a medical career instead, as she could not stand the thought of inheriting the *family traditions*.

Olivia also reported having a half-sister (from her father's side) 10 years her senior, who died of an epileptic seizure when Olivia was only 6 and once again she reported very little memories from her or the period following her death. In fact, Olivia emphasised that the only connection she had with her half-sister was through a family album and stories she heard about her, without any real affective or mnemonic account of her own. Her half-sister did not live in the family home and this is how Olivia explained the gap in her memory.

As an adult, Olivia consumed herself in short-term romantic relationships with 'handsome and high-status' men, but struggled to form intimate bonds reporting a feeling of suffocation and an aversion to co-dependency. She never married or had children, lived on her own and was fully dedicated to her career. Despite her professional success, social recognition and physical attractiveness, Olivia reported a chronic sense of emptiness, prolonged melancholia that was only interrupted by long-haul vocational activities, and a bizarre sense that she was fundamentally unloved. While she enjoyed conquering and dominating her lovers sexually, she reported episodes of anorgasmia (which she would also hide well in an attempt to get her lovers' complete surrender to her sexual charisma and achieve a narcissistic triumph).

More recently, she disclosed that she always had moments of silent crying during sexual intercourse that she would master by ending these relationships before they would develop into something more meaningful. Olivia sought therapy mainly to target her substance misuse as she became acutely aware that the use of heroin was serving a self-preservatory purpose that instinctively began to feel at odds with the causes of her existence. Olivia always maintained that she never suffered any trauma or abuse as a child, and became curious herself about the psychological origins of her long-term battle with addiction.

While Olivia struggled with her immediate recollection of her childhood memories, the material that we held was enough to explore the function of heroin as an object relation that would perform the soothing and self-regulatory functions the internalised object failed to successfully perform [33, 34]. Attending to her insecure attachment style and her relationship with her mother in particular, led us to identify Olivia's unmet narcissistic needs as a child, in terms of self-object experiences [35] and how heroin would offer her the emotional tranquillity that she was so desperate for, but unable to provide to herself as an adult, in the same way the internalised mother failed to meet her child ego's empathic needs.

Davies and Frawley assert that the traumatised child's loss of a secure base may constitute *the most pernicious and damaging psychological trauma*. Because clients' internal worlds contain partial or no representations of loving, protective objects, they never fully develop the capacity for self-soothing and self-calming at times of distress or for containment of the anxious states, disorganisation, and intense hyperarousal [37]. Relatedly, growing up with a depressed mother, Olivia's main endeavour was to save her from her demonic occupations assuming the role of the hero (often successfully as that kept her mother going) but at the expense of establishing a coherent sense of self with an *idealised internal other*. Not being able to idealise a depressed and miserable mother, Olivia had no hero for herself and *heroine* by virtue of name and quality, symbolically satisfied that unmet narcissistic need for her [35].

Attending to this transference dynamic and interpreting the re-enactment within our relationship were paramount to the healing process. Olivia would often become acutely aware of any signs of vulnerability in me, and her immediate reaction would often involve some type of kind offer to enquire into my own shortcomings (Much of those offers were products of the transference in fantasy, in the absence of any real vulnerability on my part.) I often hypothesised whether she initially aspired to become a heart surgeon because she wanted to fix the mother's heart and gain the love she was so desperate for. Olivia related to this interpretation well, noting the unconscious motivation behind the choice of her medical speciality, but she equally reported feeling loved by the mother despite her somewhat traumatic attachment to her. Rescue fantasies often occur as a result of parentification in childhood and are frequently repeated in adult relations where individuals enact the role of the hero in an attempt to achieve a narcissistic triumph and maintain the conditions of love they were initially subjected to, during childhood [35]. Rescue fantasies, however, also serve to unconsciously disavow the intolerable vulnerability of the wounded child's ego state and aspire to create a dynamic where the rescued object is finally well enough to serve their own needs (representing the weak parent in the transference).

Winnicott captured the tremendous essence of growing up with a depressed mother in his poem 'The tree', where he illustrated the intricacies of the development of the false self. Indeed, Olivia struggled with her true self expressions in all facades of her adult life and emphasised how she would receive a sense of narcissistic gratification by being admired at work, saving her patients and being desired by men, but she never managed to feel loved for who she truly was. The therapeutic space acted as a new maternal, holding environment, and during the process, we utilised Kohut's ideas of empathic resonance and attunement as the therapist's primary mode of listening, and a focus on affect as an essential component of Olivia's internal experience, which gradually aided her to build a more coherent sense of self that strengthened her capacity not only to mentalise but also tolerate her own emotional states (previously 'anesthetised' by heroin). This was accompanied by a reduction in the use of heroin and a stable compliance with her methadone schedule.

By the second year of treatment, Olivia had already managed to maintain a stable drug-free regime and demonstrated a better capacity to regulate her affective experiences, despite relying on methadone and occasionally on legal anxiolytics. However, the relinquishment of her dependency from the drug unveiled Olivia's core traumatic depression, and while her feelings of emptiness lessened, her sense of reported 'unlovability' became so raw that drove Olivia to form even more intense and rough sexual encounters whose only aim was pure libidinal gratification. It was almost as if an invisible force compelled her to seek immediate and unnegotiable physical proximity. But while she would report momentary narcissistic satisfaction from her lovers' surrender to her physical tricks, all attempts at intimacy from prospective partners were met with what she termed 'terror' and an ensuing frantic escape into a schizoid retreat. In 'a moment of meeting' [14] with Olivia, I captured her desperation inside of me in the countertransference, which I only released when I declared the annulment of all of my previous interpretations regarding the unconscious motivation behind her intense sexual activity in the absence of attachment. *Olivia was not seeking to receive love per se to satisfy a deficit in erotic resources, Olivia was seeking to grant love driven by an erotic surplus, in an attempt to re-unite with the lost object and secure her existence.*

Love has been at the heart of philosophy, psychology and psychoanalysis since conception, but sadly often trivialised by contemporaries, due to the emphasis either on the individual's *libidinal urges* as core motivators of mental life, or *relational drives* to secure survival. However, a distinguishing feature of the psychoanalytic approach is the awareness of the link between adult love and love in infancy [29].

Freud, cited in [29] postulated two models of libidinal relation—the initial narcissistic love of the ego (e.g., the mirror image sought in the other) and the anaclitic love of the object (e.g., the image of a parent). It could be argued that both types of love are anaclitic in nature as the individual requires mnemonic access to earlier patterns of relating to self and others for the repetition to occur, either pre-consciously or unconsciously. In 1912, Freud referred to love as an *affectionate current* akin to long-term attachment and differentiated it from sexual desire, which he referred to as a *sexual current*—both referring to a propelling, dynamic energy in the psyche. According to Freud, the split between *affection* and *desire* is experienced unconsciously in order to defend against punitive parental introjects, which are awakened by the experience of a new desired object in a sexually similar way as the subject felt towards the desired parent in childhood [39]. Freud referred to this as the *mother-whore* complex in male love, to illustrate the inability to maintain sexual arousal within a committed, loving relationship. This is, however, true for all relations. Clients with this complex desire a sexual partner who has been degraded, while they cannot desire the respected partner: *where such men love they have no desire and where they desire they cannot love* [38]. The person then develops two specific self-protective unconscious defences:

a. The first is an ascetic attitude towards desired objects in which disgust and humiliation are subliminally employed to thwart self-expansive, romantic urges.

b. The second is a moral masochistic reaction of guilt in the wake of desire. The person unwittingly assumes that yearning for new objects of desire is an act of disloyalty to parental introjects. To avoid this primal sin, the person seeks to evoke rejecting responses from the desired object by pushing them away. Interpersonal hurt then disrupts the transfer of incestuous impulses from a parental introject onto the new object. According to Freud, to defend against additional infantile patterns—repressive, seductive, magical longings for the 'lost' object of the parent–child bonding—moral masochism and asceticism work together, alternating in dominance [38].

In Olivia's case, however, the process of erotic connection with the potential of leading to deeper intimacy was evoked by the thwarting of her own loving urges—not her partners' evoked rejection, who on the contrary demonstrated an eager and often affectionate attitude towards her. In fact, Olivia's attraction would immediately cease once the desired lover would attempt to transform into an affectionate partner.

Secondly, Olivia's comfort with sexual proximity was anything but ascetic. Her compulsive hyperarousal, in fact, served to enhance the split between affection and desire in as much as desire for anonymous objects (short-term flings) would compensate for the lack of affection for an eponymous subject (long-term, stable attachments). The wake of the potential of affection towards an admirable and respected partner seemed to overwhelm her ego, sending her into a one-way schizoid retreat. Fairbairn observed that the schizoid's main conflict lied in the individual's perception of their own love as 'bad' and Olivia's moral masochism manifested in the halting of her own expressions of affection towards the subject, not the other way round.

The next logical question was 'why'. There was nothing in Olivia's narrative that would point to an earlier oedipal, traumatic experience that would account for the internalisation of her own love as destructive. I had already attempted to make a link between her father's absence and her avoidant attachment style, which could have in part explained her distaste of bonds, but Olivia did not react with any substantial insight into that either. Having no material to work with from her earlier history and being confronted with Olivia's severe depression, left me with no choice but to attend to her current acting out as the last resort to make sense of her suffering. Olivia continued to report outbursts of silent crying during sexual intercourse and affirmed her feelings of 'terror' every time a prospective lover invited her to reciprocate love in the form of relational affection—that is, every time the erotic physical yearning threatened to become an erotic relation.

During the later stages of treatment and while following this line of enquiry, Olivia met an older man who fell in love with her and resisted her continuous rejections by persevering into creating a long-term relationship with her. Olivia's depression worsened over the coming weeks and she eventually relapsed into heroin, and suffered a myocardial infraction. Her heart was about to stop and she would no longer be confronted with the pain of needing to give love—the ghost of her unspent love would be long gone.

Olivia suffered a heart attack on the grounds of a hospital a few minutes before she was due to start work and was found immediately by a fellow doctor who proceeded to transfer her to the emergency room for resuscitation and emergency angioplasty. When she returned to therapy 6 weeks later, Olivia reported the following experience:

Following the coronary angioplasty and during the process of arousal from the general anaesthesia, Olivia entered a semi-conscious state where she began to recount memories from her childhood. This continued throughout her recovery process in the coming weeks where she was bombarded with lucid images from her past. Olivia recalled herself as a child visiting her half-sister's house with her father, where she would be left to play on her own in the garden, while he would spend time indoors with the half-sister. Olivia recalled herself looking through the glass door into the living room and seeing images of her half-sister who was a teenager at the time, entering vague sexual encounters with the father. At the time, none of the scattered nude images or their proximal physical postures arising from gaps in the curtains made sense to her but evoked a strong feeling of terror. Olivia also remembered hearing her half-sister declaring her love for him on numerous other occasions and him demonstrating a bizarre, adoring attachment towards her. Olivia remembered attempting to ask her father about physical love between people and being heavily reprimanded for making such unacceptable enquiries. Olivia remembered feeling scared but forming a clear understanding at the age of 6, of what Eros meant, and what falling in love feels like. Olivia remembered sensing a confusing arousal inside her 6-year-old body—a precocious maturity. Olivia remembered telling her mother that she was scared of the father and her mother dismissing her. Olivia remembered that her half-sister died suddenly of an epileptic fit and that her father entered an inconsolable depression after that. Olivia remembered her father travelling abroad all the time following the death and being completely absent from her life. During his inconsistent returns home, Olivia remembered her father visiting her bedroom after midnight and her whole body shaking with terror, freezing into the foetal position. Olivia did not remember any sexual encounter with the father she admired, respected and loved, but remembered picturing the full meaning of love:death. Olivia painted many pictures of lovers that die in lust, at her after-school painting club, which she would often erase using white spirit.

4.2 Discussion and outcome

In the proceeding sessions, it was made clear that Olivia's trauma had been dissociated from her conscious mind but fully absorbed and acted out in child play, in her behaviour towards adult relations, in her belief system and in her attachment style. Ferenczi illustrated how sexually traumatised clients may have little if any memory of the event largely due to the disbelief, minimization, and denial exhibited by adults in the child's environment, whenever efforts were made to introduce the topic of seduction. In tandem with the child's desire to maintain some sort of loving connection with the parents, these reactions are further reason for the child to disbelieve their own veridical recollections and to conclude that the seduction imagined was simply a fantasy production [14]. However, the memory of the veritable seduction experience and the resultant trauma do remain, creating a fragmented personality, in a way that each split or division in the personality behaves as though *it does not know of the existence of the others*. According to Ringel and Blandell ([14], p. 45) *what is especially remarkable about this portrayal is how well it resonates with contemporary psychological formulations of the processes and phenomena of dissociation, now universally recognized as a hallmark of the post-traumatic adaptation* [14].

For Olivia, the operation of dissociation primarily allowed her to tolerate the reality of the distressing event by splitting off highly incoherent or overwhelming thoughts, memories and feelings [29, 32, 37] associated with witnessing her half-sister's incestuous relationship with the father. The task of therapy was to help her integrate these memories into her personality while increasing her capacity to tolerate and process the affects and interpretations associated with the traumatic experience. Ringel and Blandell [14] quote Davies and Frawley who noted that *with no self-reflective observing ego to provide even the rudiments of containment, meaning and structure to the traumatic events, the child exists in a timeless, objectless and selfless nightmare of unending pain, isolation and ultimately, psychic dissolution* (p. 75). According to the authors, it is not just the traumatic memories that become dissociated from other experiences but also *the organization of mutually exclusive systems of self and object representation*s (p. 75) formed in relation to traumatic experiences. The therapeutic process, as a result, must achieve integration not only of the memories themselves but also of clients' varying experiences of self in relation to their fragmented worlds of internal objects [14].

The concept of enactment was necessary and instrumental in Olivia's treatment outcome in as much as it offered us a platform to observe the unconscious repetition of her primary relational and intrapsychic conflict, which led to the eventual dissolution of the dissociation and her successful abreaction of the trauma. As mentioned above, a central conundrum of Olivia's traumatic depression was the split between her sexual behaviour and her attachment system—a dichotomy between desire and affection. Olivia seemed to have internalised a very antithetical vision of her father both as an oedipal object of desire, and as an attachment figure of resourcefulness and *potential* security. Witnessing the sexual incest and the simultaneous enmeshing attachment between her half-sister and her father, which was eventually interrupted by her death, led Olivia to develop a series of fantasies associated with her own capacity to express sexual desire and loving affection. In the final stages of treatment, Olivia was able to articulate how love, both in the form of affection and desire, threatened to bring about some sort of disaster (i.e., psychical death) in the same fashion her half-sister died for entertaining both internal states. Moreover, her father's subsequent distant attitude led her to fear the consequences of her own affectional loving urges (possibly by introjecting his own incestuous guilt) and the safest way to prevent the impending catastrophe was to keep desire and affection separate. However, her compulsive urges to enter intense sexual relations were a reminder of her own uninvested or unspent love, and her failure to achieve a satisfactory outcome in terms of developing a lasting relational bond was possibly the most alerting signal of the enormity of her dual conflict: the intrapsychic vs. the interpersonal. According to Eagle ([39], p. 221) *One classic and primary expression of an inadequately resolved Oedipal conflict is a relative inability to integrate sexual and lustful feelings on the one hand and tender and loving feelings on the other, that is, to have both sets of feelings towards the same person. One consequence of such an unresolved conflict, which often brings people into treatment, is great difficulty in establishing and maintaining long-lasting intimate relationships*.

The relationship between sexuality and attachment is not fully understood yet but contemporary theorists have attempted to shed some light on it by presenting it mainly as a parallel and antagonistic process facilitated by two distinct subsystems [40, 41] or as intertwined co-occurring systems that require integration for patients who might have suffered trauma [42]. The latter seems to be a more plausible explanation of the processes of attachment and sexuality in trauma, as the complete separation of the two, admits to a number of limitations, which go beyond the scope of this chapter. Eagle [41] supported the view that attachment and sexuality are functionally separable systems and, in certain respects, operate in mutually antagonistic ways. He further proposed that the integration of attachment and sexuality is a developmental challenge that is met by different people with varying degrees of success depending, in part, upon their individual attachment pattern. With regard to Freud's postulation of moral masochism stemming from incestuous longings, Eagle correctly argued that whereas an incest taboo is relevant to understanding the split between love and desire, there is little evidence that universal incestuous wishes play a central role in accounting for that phenomenon [41]. Holmes [39] noted that it is not uncommon for partners to be intensely attached to each other with a relative absence of sexual interest and conversely that sexual involvement may preclude an attachment relationship. Fonagy also remarked that that these systems are separate and at most loosely coupled [39]. Diamond emphasised this separation by noting that *desire is governed by the sexual mating system* (p. 174), the goal of which is reproduction, whereas love *is governed by the attachment or pair-bonding system...the goal of which is the maintenance of an enduring association* (p. 174) for the purpose of survival of dependent offspring [43].

While these observations hold tremendous theoretical value, they do not account fully for the intertwining between the two, given that Eros does not necessarily aspire to reproduction, but to other forms of connection including intimacy and unity. The latter is especially true for same-sex desire where the innate reproduction code is intact, but does not drive sexual longing *per se*. Kirkpatrick pointed out that the need for intimacy seems to be greater among women than men in homo-erotic relationships, and that genital release may not be their primary organising and motivating factor.

Moreover, we do not hold sufficient research outcomes to validate the claim that some sexual relations do not involve an attachment relationship at all. It may well be the case that the attachment dynamic is dominated by distance and minimisation, in which case we might be dealing with a biphasic defensive operation of symbolic character, rather than a complete lack of connection between lovers. Sexual arousal is indeed heightened by unfamiliar, distant and mystic attractions, but this may not necessarily preclude the undercurrent of attachment—in fact, examining the phantasies of the object representation may have a lot to say about the nature of these psychosexual dynamics beyond pure instinctual organisation.

Eagle [41] noted that with regard to the transference dynamic, the more unresolved one's early attachment relationship, which is characteristic of insecure attachment, the more one will react to current partner as a stand-in for a parent, and the less able one will be to experience one's current partner as a sexual figure. *That one continues to be avoidant toward current partner strongly suggests that one is continuing to react defensively, as if one were experiencing current partner as rejecting and/or intrusive, similar to the way one experienced the early parental figure* [41].

Olivia's traumatic depression was reinforced by her dissociation, concealed by her substance misuse and further elaborated by her inability to invest her loving urges towards potential partners, because attachment was equated with death in fantasy. The same did not apply to her sexuality though, apart from her chronic anorgasmia, which was another symptom of her traumatic exposure.

During the final stages of treatment, we focused on creating a more coherent narrative of her traumatic past, developed a new template of object-relations where love would meet desire in a non-destructive manner characterised by integration of the two; while allowing her to build a more stable sense of self that inclined her to attempt something a bit more meaningful with her partner than raw sex.

Davies and Frawley [37] strongly endorse the therapeutic relationship for acting as a vehicle through, which 'soothing, undoing and redoing' of the traumatised client's life must finally occur largely based on the therapist's 'willingness to know' the person fully. The relational model composed of various psychoanalytic contributions emphasises the intersubjective dynamics between client and, important others as well as client and therapist, around interpersonal enactments stemming from the traumatic experience. Enactments are seen not only as essential but also as instrumental in helping clients process and make sense of the previously unconscious relational patterns that they find themselves in, their impact on self and others, and their perception and interpretation of others' words and behaviours.

5. Epilogue: *To love is to give what one does not have*

Studies of traumatised children have demonstrated unequivocally that infants and toddlers have the prerequisite emotional and cognitive capacities for trauma to have persisting effects on their psyche. Traumatised children can retain some type of internal representation of their trauma for years, as demonstrated through trauma-centric behavioural re-enactments, affective responses to traumatic triggers, expressive play, sensory and somatic symptoms, and even verbal recall [44].

Historically, a conception that has had wide currency within the psychodynamic school of thought is that psychological trauma in childhood both interrupts development and scars it forever. The overwhelming of the ego induced by psychological trauma is theorised to exert enduring memory imprints that cause intrusive flashbacks, emotional re-experiencing, traumatically driven behavioural re-enactments, trauma-centric fears, and disturbing dreams [20–26, 42].

The trauma is seen as having an enduring organisational influence on the client throughout the life span, a conception Gaensbauer and Jordan termed as a 'full-fledged' repetition. Analysing cases of traumatised adults and children, Herman ([24], p.32) concluded that *long after the trauma is past, traumatized people relive the event as though it were continually recurring in the present...the traumatic moment becomes encoded...and breaks spontaneously into consciousness, both as flashbacks during waking states and as traumatic nightmares during sleep* [24, 44]. Olivia's traumatic depression lied in the early sexual trauma she was exposed to and although she did not have any recollections of being sexually abused herself, the enormity of the terror she witnessed damaged her developmental potential and the capacity to form healthy relationships driven by a constant battle between desire and affection towards an object that held oppositional qualities; a battle of gifting love driven by a lack of security. Lacan's famous aphorism on love was *loving is to give what one does not have.* For Lacan, this is the essence of loving—the key to love, to being able to love, is to accept one's lack: *One cannot love except by becoming a non-haver, even if one has* [45].

Conflict of interest

The author declares no conflict of interest.

Author details

Catherine Athanasiadou-Lewis
Department of Psychology, London Metropolitan University, London, England

*Address all correspondence to: c.athanasiadoulewis@londonmet.ac.uk

References

[1] McCarthy J. A framework for healing from loss: A further integration of psychodynamic and social work theory. Journal of Human Behavior in the Social Environment. 2006;**14**:45-79

[2] Kalsched D. The Inner World of Trauma: Archetypal Defenses of the Personal Spirit. London/New York: Routledge; 1996

[3] Greening T. PTSD from the perspective of existential-humanistic psychology. Journal of Traumatic Stress. 1990;**3**(2):323-326

[4] Lazaratou H. Interpersonal trauma: Psychodynamic psychotherapy and neurobiology. European Journal of Psychotraumatology. 2017;**8**(4):135202. DOI: 10.1080/20008198.2017.1351202

[5] Pearlman L, Saakvitne K. Trauma and the therapist: Countertransference and vicarious traumatization in psychotherapy with incest survivors. The American Journal of Clinical Hypnosis. 1995;**38**(4):298-299. DOI: 10.1080/00029157.1996.10403354

[6] Allen J. Coping with Trauma: A Guide to Self-Understanding. Washington, DC: American Psychiatric Press; 1995

[7] Jackowski A, De Araújo C, De Lacerda A, De Jesus M, Kaufman J. Neurostructural imaging findings in children with post-traumatic stress disorder: Brief review. Psychiatry and Clinical Neurosciences. 2009;**63**(1):1-8

[8] Schore A. Relational trauma and the developing right brain. Self and Systems: Annals of New York Academic Sciences. 2009;**1159**:189-203. DOI: 10.1111/j.1749-6632.2009.04474

[9] Fine C. The tactical-integration model for the treatment of dissociative identity disorder and allied dissociative disorders. American Journal of Psychotherapy. 1999;**53**(3):361-376

[10] Lineham M, Tutek D, Heard H, Armstrong H. Interpersonal outcome of cognitive behavioral treatment for chronically suicidal borderline patients. The American Journal of Psychiatry. 1994;**151**(12):1771-1776

[11] Shapiro F. EMDR treatment: Overview and integration. In: Shapiro F, editor. EMDR as an Integrative Psychotherapy Approach: Experts of Diverse Orientations Explore the Paradigm Prism. Washington, DC: American Psychological Association; 2002. pp. 27-55

[12] Westen D, Novotny C, Thompson-Brenner H. The empirical status of empirically supported psychotherapies: Assumptions, findings, and reporting in controlled clinical trials. Psychological Bulletin. 2004;**130**(4):631-663

[13] Sachsse U, Vogel C, Leichsenring F. Results of psychodynamically oriented trauma-focussed inpatient treatment for women with complex posttraumatic stress disorder (PTSD) and borderline personality diosrder (BPD). Bulletin of the Menninger Clinic. 2006;**70**(2):125-144

[14] Ringel S, Blandell J. Trauma: Contemporary Directions in Theory, Practice, and Research. London: Sage; 2012

[15] van der Kolk B, Pelcovitz D, Roth S, Mandel F, McFarlane A, Herman J. Dissociation, somatization, and affect dysregulation: The complexity of adaptation to trauma. The American Journal of Psychiatry. 1996;**153**(7):83-93

[16] Halewood A. Psychodynamic counselling psychology. In: Murphy D,

editor. Counselling Psychology: A Textbook for Study and Practice. 1st ed. London: Willey and Sons; 2017. pp. 89-103

[17] Kardiner A. The Traumatic Neuroses of War. New York: Hoerber; 1941

[18] van der Kolk B, McFarlane A, Weisaeth L, editors. Traumatic Stress: The Effects of Overwhelming Experience on Mind, Body and Society. 1st ed. New York: Guilford; 1996

[19] Athanasiadou-Lewis C. A critical evaluation of the conceptual model and empirical evidence for current cognitive behavioral approaches to post-traumatic stress disorder from a counseling psychology perspective. Edorium Journal of Psychology. 2017;**3**:1-9

[20] McNally R. The ontology of posttraumatic stress disorder: Natural kind, social construction, or causal system? Clinical Psychology: Science and Practice. 2012;**19**:220-229

[21] Young A. The Harmony of Illusions: Inventing Posttraumatic Stress Disorder. Princeton, NJ: Princeton University Press; 1995

[22] Yehuda R, McFarlane A. Conflict between current knowledge about posttraumatic stress disorder and its original conceptual basis. The American Journal of Psychiatry. 1995;**152**:1705-1713

[23] Chertoff J. Psychodynamic assessment and treatment of traumatized patients. The Journal of Psychotherapy Practice and Research. 1998;**7**:35-46

[24] Herman J. Complex PTSD: A syndrome in survivors of prolonged and repeated trauma. Journal of Traumatic Stress. 1992;**5**:377-391

[25] Ford J, Courtois C. Defining and understanding complex trauma and complex traumatic stress disorders. In: Courtois A, Ford J, editors. Treating Complex Traumatic Stress Disorders: An Evidence-Based Guide. 1st ed. New York: Guilford Press; 2009. pp. 13-30

[26] Schottenbauer M, Glass C, Diane B, Arnkoff B, Hafter Gray S. Contributions of psychodynamic approaches to treatment of PTSD and trauma: A review of the empirical treatment and psychopathology literature. Psychiatry. 2008;**7**:23-34

[27] Freud S. The ego and the id. In: Strachey J, editor. The Standard Edition of the Complete Psychological Works of Sigmund Freud. London: Hogarth Press; 1961. pp. 1-66

[28] Lacewing M. Love, Reality and Psychoanalysis [Internet]. 2019. Available from: https://sas-space.sas.ac.uk/730/1/M_Lacewing_Love.pdf

[29] Fenichel O. The Psychoanalytic Theory of Neurosis. New York: W.W Norton; 1996

[30] Freud S. 'Remembering,' 'Repeating' and 'Working-Through' (Further Recommendations on the Technique of Psycho-Analysis II). In: Strachey J, editor. The Standard Edition of the Complete Psychological Works of Sigmund Freud. London: Hogarth Press; 1958. pp. 145-147

[31] Mitchell S, Black M. Freud and Beyond: A History of Modem Psychoanalytic Thought. New York: Basic Books; 1995

[32] Ferenczi S. The confusion of tongues between adults and the child: The language of tenderness and passion. In: Balint M, Mosbacher E, et al., editors. Final Contributions to the Problems and Methods of

Psyho-Analysis. London: Karnac Books; 1980. pp. 156-167

[33] Winnicott D. The theory of the parent-infant relationship. In: Buckley P, editor. Essential Papers in Psychoanalysis. Essential Papers on Object Relations. New York, NY, USA: New York University Press; 1986

[34] Winnicott D. Ego Distortion in Terms of True and False Self. The Maturational Process and the Facilitating Environment. New York: International Universities Press; 1960. pp. 140-152

[35] Kohut H. The Restoration of the Self. New York: International Universities Press; 1977

[36] Fonagy P, Target M. Attachment and reflective function: Their role in self-organization. Development and Psychopathology. 1997;**9**:679-700

[37] Davies J, Frawley M. Treating the Adult Survivor of Childhood Sexual Abuse: A Psychoanalytic Perspective. New York: Basic Books; 1994

[38] Goldberg C. A psychoanalysis of love: The patient with deadly longing. American Journal of Psychotherapy. 1999;**3**:437-451

[39] Eagle M. Attachment and psychoanalysis. The British Journal of Medical Psychology. 1997;**70**:217-229

[40] Diamond D, Blatt S, Lichtenberg J, editors. Psychoanalytic Inquiry Book Series: Vol. 21. Attachment and Sexuality. New York, NY, USA: The Analytic Press/ Taylor & Francis Group; 2007

[41] Eagle M. Attachment and sexuality. In: Diamond D, Blatt S, Lichtenberg J, editors. Psychoanalytic Inquiry Book Series: Vol. 21. Attachment and Sexuality. New York, NY, USA: The Analytic Press/ Taylor & Francis Group; 2007

[42] Stefanou C, McCabe M. Adult attachment and sexual functioning: A review of past research. The Journal of Sexual Medicine. 2012;**9**(10):2499-2507

[43] Diamond L. What does sexual orientation orient? A biobehavioral model in distinguishng romantic love and sexual desire. Psycho-logical Review. 2003;**110**(1):173-192

[44] Gaensbauer T, Jordan L. Psychoanalytic perspectives on early trauma: Interviews with thirty analysts who treated an adult victim of a circumscribed trauma in early childhood. Journal of the American Psychoanalytic Association. 2009;**57**:947. DOI: 10.1177/0003065109342589

[45] Miller J, editor. The Seminars of Jacques Lacan Book XIII: Transference, 1961-1962. Cambridge: Polity; 2015

Chapter 3

Eicosapentaenoic Acid Intake Associated with Reduced Risk of Posttraumatic Stress Disorder after the Great East Japan Earthquake and Tsunami

Emiko Aizawa, Miho Ota, Ikki Ishida, Norie Koga, Kotaro Hattori, Shinji Sato, Takashi Asada and Hiroshi Kunugi

Abstract

Posttraumatic stress disorder (PTSD) is a debilitating condition characterized by intrusion, avoidance, hyperarousal symptoms after exposure to traumatic events. Since polyunsaturated fatty acids (PUFAs) have been implicated, we examined the possible association of PTSD with plasma PUFA level and dietary fish intake in 563 women who was struck by the Great East Japan Earthquake and Tsunami. The impact event scale-revised (IES-R) was used to assess PTSD symptoms. Dietary intake was estimated by a self-report questionnaire. Multivariate analysis controlling for age, body mass index, and stress revealed that PTSD status (IES-R $\geq$ 25) was associated with plasma eicosapentaenoic acid (EPA) level (P = 0.039). In the high-stress group, there were significantly inverse correlations of plasma EPA with IES-R total (r = −0.389, P = 0.031), intrusion (r = −0.370, P = 0.04), and hyperarousal scores (r = −0.480, P = 0.006), although such correlations were not found in the moderate-stress group. Fish intake that increased plasma EPA showed similar correlations with IES-R scores in the severely stressed group. Our results suggest that higher plasma EPA level and EPA-increasing fish intake are associated with a lower risk for PTSD in individuals who have suffered severe stress in a natural disaster.

Keywords: posttraumatic stress disorder, Great East Japan Earthquake, eicosapentaenoic acid, nutrition

1. Introduction

Posttraumatic stress disorder (PTSD) is a debilitating psychiatric condition characterized by intrusion, avoidance, hyperarousal, and other symptoms, which occurs in response to an array of traumatic events including physical, sexual, or mental abuse; wartime experiences; or being the victim of a violent crime [1]. The resulting stress can cause a pro-inflammatory response in the brain characterized primarily by the complex release of inflammatory mediators such as cytokines, prostanoids, free radicals, and transcription factors, as well as subsequent brain inflammatory responses, which further contribute to cell damage [2, 3]. Conventional treatment for PTSD includes pharmacotherapy, psychotherapy, and psychophysiological therapy, although it is often resistant to these treatments [4].

An alternative strategy might be the use of diet or nutritional care, particularly those focusing on polyunsaturated fatty acids (PUFAs) such as eicosapentaenoic acid (EPA; C20: 5n-3), docosahexaenoic acid (DHA; C22: 6n-3), and arachidonic acid (AA; C20: 4n-6) in preventing and treating PTSD [5]. A series of studies by Matsuoka and colleagues [6–9] reported that the effect of DHA on the prevention of PTSD was minimal; however, subsequent elevation of EPA level in erythrocytes was correlated with less PTSD symptoms and better quality of life. However, there is a dearth of studies on the possible relationship between blood levels of PUFAs and the risk of PTSD. The same research group found that AA and EPA levels in the serum were both inversely related to the risk for PTSD in subjects of post-motor vehicle accident [10]. Kalinic et al. reported inverse correlations of EPA, but not AA or DHA, levels in the serum with the severity of combat-related PTSD symptoms in Croatian war veterans [11]. These results were, at least in part, inconsistent, which requires further investigations.

In the present study, we examined the relationships of plasma levels and dietary intake of PUFAs with the development of PTSD among women who lived in Kitaibaraki city and struck by the Great East Japan Earthquake and Tsunami on March 11, 2011.

2. Subjects and methods

2.1 Study population

The study population consisted of volunteers who were living in the earthquake disaster zone in Kitaibaraki, Japan, a city with a population of approximately 45,000. Our study was conducted from November 2011 to August 2012. Participants were selected based on the following criteria: females who were 20 years or older on November 1, 2011 and were able to come to a local hospital on their own. The study population was limited to females in order to eliminate the gender differences reported in the response to traumatic events [12] and in effects of PUFAs [6].

Our study population comprised 563 women (mean age: 53.3 ± 15.8). A total of 113 out of the 563 participants lived along the coastline where the impact of the tsunami was particularly high. The study was fully explained to all potential participants, after which written informed consent to the participation was obtained. This study was conducted in accordance with the declaration of Helsinki [13] and approved by the ethics committees of the University of Tsukuba and the National Center of Neurology and Psychiatry, Japan.

2.2 Dividing the study population into four groups

The study population was then ultimately divided into four groups through a two-stage process: first determining stress exposure and second determining the presence of PTSD. Participants were initially asked to fill out an original four-item questionnaire developed by our group. This questionnaire is designed to assess the degree of exposure to stress caused by the earthquake and tsunami and provide a total impact score. These four items inquired the occurrence of: (1) severe injury or death among close relatives (one point per person), (2) severe inundation-related damage to house or apartment of the participant, (3) partial or complete destruction of a housing unit and/or household belongings, and (4) significant decrease in income. The study population was then divided into a high stress group and moderate stress group based on the results of the questionnaire. The high stress group was defined as including participants who were impacted by three or more of the abovementioned items. The moderate stress group was defined as those participants who were impacted by two or less of the items.

Next, these high-stress and moderate-stress groups were each further divided into two groups: those participants with PTSD (PTSD group) and those without PTSD (non-PTSD group) based on the IES-R questionnaire. **Figure 1** shows the numbers of individuals for the four groups of high-stress/PTSD, high-stress/non-PTSD, moderate-stress/PTSD, and moderate-stress/non-PTSD.

2.3 IES-R questionnaire

The Japanese version of IES-R questionnaire was used to screen for PTSD symptoms because IES-R is the most widely used questionnaire in all forms of disaster-area research [14, 15]. This questionnaire consists of 22 items that comprise three subscales of intrusion (8 items), avoidance (8 items), and hyperarousal (6 items). IES-R evaluates symptom severity using a 5-point scale (0–4) for the previous 1-week period. PTSD was defined as present when the IES-R score was 25 or more, according to a previous study [16].

2.4 Assessment of dietary intake

Dietary intake was assessed using the brief-type self-administered diet history questionnaire (BDHQ) [17, 18]. This questionnaire assesses diet habits in the preceding month. Dietary intake, particularly fish intake, was calculated using an *ad hoc* computer algorithm (including weighting factors) designed specifically for the BDHQ. Dietary intake was adjusted by using the nutrient density method defined as the percentage of energy for energy-providing nutrients and amount per 1000 kcal of energy for other nutrients. In BDHQ, fish intake was assessed by six categories: category 1 (C1): squid, shrimp, lobster, and shellfish; C2: whole-eat fish; C3: canned tuna; C4: dried fish/salted fish; C5: oil-rich fish; and C6: non-oil-rich fish.

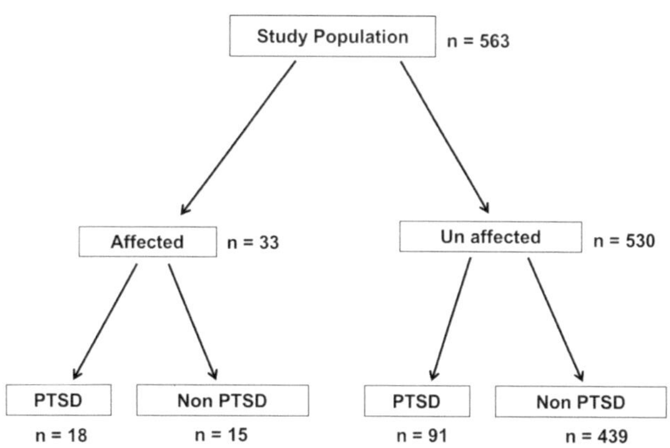

Figure 1.
Diagram of data analysis procedure. The study population was divided into four groups through a two-stage process: first by determining stress exposure and second by determining the presence of PTSD.

2.5 Measurement of plasma fatty acids

Non-fasting venous blood samples were collected between the hours of 9:00 and 15:00 from each participant to determine the plasma levels of EPA, DHA, and AA. These samples were collected in tubes containing ethylenediaminetetraacetic acid (EDTA) and were centrifuged at 3000*g* for 10 min. Plasma fatty acids were measured by gas chromatography (Gas Chromatograph, Model GC-2010, Shimadzu Corporation, Japan) [19] at the SRL Inc. (Tokyo Japan).

2.6 Statistical analysis

Participant characteristics, biochemical, and nutritional data are presented as mean ± standard deviation (SD) or the number of persons. Analysis of variance (ANOVA) was used to examine differences in demographic and clinical variables between the high-stress and moderate-stress groups as well as between the PTSD and non-PTSD groups. The X^2 test for independence was used to compare the prevalence of PTSD between high- and moderate-stress groups. Differences in values between PTSD and non-PTSD were examined for the blood test results and nutrients assessed by BDHQ using two-way multiple analysis of covariance (MANCOVA) after adjustment for age and body mass index (BMI). Partial correlation analysis adjusting for age and BMI was used to examine relationships of plasma EPA level and fish intake with IES-R scores. Analysis was performed using the Statistical Package for the Social Sciences (SPSS) version 21.0 (SPSS Japan, Tokyo). Statistical significance was set at two-tailed $P < 0.05$.

3. Results

3.1 Characteristics of the study participants

The characteristics of the study participants are shown for the high- and moderate-stress groups after each group was further divided into PTSD and non-PTSD groups (**Table 1**). No significant differences were found in age, BMI, or education between the high- and moderate-stress groups or between the PTSD and non-PTSD groups. As expected, the degree of exposure to stress of the high-stress group was significantly higher than moderate-stress group. The prevalence of PTSD was 55% for the high stress group and 17% for the moderate stress group [$X^2 = 27.8$, df = 1, $P = 0.00000013$, Cramer's V = 0.22, odds ratio; 5.8, 95% confidence interval (CI): 2.8–11.9]. As expected, the PTSD group exhibited significantly higher scores for the total IES-R score as well as the intrusion, avoidance, and hyperarousal subscales than the non-PTSD group.

3.2 Association between plasma EPA level and PTSD

Plasma PUFA concentrations for the four groups are shown in **Table 2**. MANCOVA analysis controlling for age and BMI revealed that PTSD was significantly associated with plasma EPA level [$F(1, 557) = 4.27$, $P = 0.039$, partial $\eta^2 = 0.008$], but not with DHA [$F(1, 557) = 1.98$, $P = 0.16$, partial $\eta^2 = 0.004$], or AA [$F(1, 557) = 0.186$, $P = 0.174$, partial $\eta^2 = 0.003$] and that there was a non-significant association between PTSD and EPA/AA ratio [$F(1, 557) = 3.28$, $P = 0.071$, partial $\eta^2 = 0.006$]. It also detected a stress × PTSD interaction effect on plasma EPA level at a trend level [$F(1, 557) = 3.281$, $P = 0.091$, partial $\eta^2 = 0.005$]. As shown in **Table 2**, mean plasma EPA level was substantially higher in the non-PTSD group than in the PTSD group among individuals who had high stress, while it was similar for the PTSD and non-PTSD groups among

Characteristics	High stress		Moderate stress		*F* value; partial η^2	*P* value; high stress v. moderate stress	*F* value; partial η^2	*P* value; PTSD v. non-PTSD
	PTSD ($n = 18$)	Non-PTSD ($n = 15$)	PTSD ($n = 91$)	Non-PTSD ($n = 439$)				
Age (years)	57.8 ± 14.3	57.7 ± 13.2	54.6 ± 16.7	52.7 ± 15.7	$F(1, 559) = 2.032$; partial $\eta^2 = 0.004$	0.155	$F(1, 559) = 0.111$; partial $\eta^2 = 0.000$	0.739
BMI (kg/cm^2)	24.7 ± 4.9	24.1 ± 3.6	23.6 ± 3.9	23.1 ± 3.8	$F(1, 559) = 2.204$; partial $\eta^2 = 0.004$	0.138	$F(1, 559) = 0.487$; partial $\eta^2 = 0.001$	0.486
Education (years)	12.2 ± 2.4	12.0 ± 2.2	11.4 ± 1.9	12.2 ± 2.2	$F(1, 559) = 0.626$; partial $\eta^2 = 0.001$	0.429	$F(1, 559) = 0.402$; partial $\eta^2 = 0.001$	0.526
The degree of exposure to stress								
Total points	3.1 ± 0.24	3.0 ± 0.0	1.1 ± 0.8	1.0 ± 0.7	$F(1, 559) = 240.1$; partial $\eta^2 = 0.3$	**<0.001**	$F(1, 559) = 0.644$; partial $\eta^2 = 0.001$	0.423
Death or injury in relatives, n (%)	4 (22%)	4 (27%)	4 (4%)	13 (3%)	$F(1, 559) = 45.87$; partial $\eta^2 = 0.076$	**<0.001**		0.216
Inundation damage, n (%)	14 (78%)	11 (73%)	8 (9%)	26 (6%)	$F(1, 559) = 203.1$; partial $\eta^2 = 0.266$	**<0.001**		0.445
Material damage, n (%)	18 (100%)	14 (93%)	63 (69%)	284 (64%)	$F(1, 559) = 12.1$; partial $\eta^2 = 0.021$	**0.001**		0.512
Decreased income, n (%)	18 (100%)	14 (93%)	26 (29%)	97 (22%)	$F(1, 559) = 88.3$; partial $\eta^2 = 0.004$	**<0.001**		0.387
IES-RIES-R								
IES-R score	38.8 ± 14.3	13.7 ± 6.5	37.9 ± 12.4	8.7 ± 6.8	$F(1, 559) = 3.629$; partial $\eta^2 = 0.006$	0.057	$F(1, 559) = 0.318$; partial $\eta^2 = 0.363$	**<0.001**
IES-R intrusion	14.5 ± 6.5	5.4 ± 2.7	14.3 ± 5.3	3.4 ± 3.0	$F(1, 559) = 2.647$; partial $\eta^2 = 0.005$	0.104	$F(1, 559) = 227.3$; partial $\eta^2 = 0.289$	**<0.001**

Characteristics	High stress		Moderate stress		F value; partial η^2	P value; high stress v. moderate stress	F value; partial η^2	P value; PTSD v. non-PTSD
	PTSD (n = 18)	Non-PTSD (n = 15)	PTSD (n = 91)	Non-PTSD (n = 439)				
IES-R avoidance	13.7 ± 4.9	5.4 ± 2.9	13.5 ± 4.9	3.1 ± 3.4	$F(1, 559) = 3.50$; partial $\eta^2 = 0.006$	0.062	$F(1, 559) = 182.7$; partial $\eta^2 = 0.246$	**<0.001**
IES-R hyperarousal	10.6 ± 5.2	2.9 ± 1.6	10.1 ± 4.4	2.4 ± 2.3	$F(1, 559) = 0.670$; partial $\eta^2 = 0.001$	0.414	$F(1, 559) = 214.9$; partial $\eta^2 = 0.278$	**<0.001**

P value for differences among high stress and moderate stress, as well as PTSD and non-PTSD were calculated by using analysis of variance (ANOVA). Significant results are indicated in bold letters.
Mean ± SD (standard deviation, all such values).
IES-R, impact event scale-revised.

Table 1.
Characteristics of the study participants (n = 563).

Fatty acid	High stress		Moderate stress		*F* value; partial η^2	*P*; PTSD v. non-PTSD
	PTSD (n = 18)	Non-PTSD (n = 15)	PTSD (n = 91)	Non-PTSD (n = 439)		
EPA	77.0 ± 33.5	107.4 ± 67.4	77.3 ± 43.3	76.9 ± 53.9	F(1, 559) = 4.27; partial η^2 = 0.008	0.039*
DHA	168.8 ± 41.8	191.8 ± 65.6	168.9 ± 60.5	166.5 ± 63.6	F(1, 559) = 1.98; partial η^2 = 0.004	0.160
AA	196.8 ± 49.6	207.6 ± 50.6	186.7 ± 29.3	194.1 ± 42.3	F(1, 559) = 1.86; partial η^2 = 0.003	0.174
EPA/AA	2.40 ± 1.19	3.41 ± 2.06	2.45 ± 1.66	2.48 ± 1.94	F(1, 559) = 3.28; partial η^2 = 0.006	0.071

AA, arachidonic acid; EPA, eicosapentaenoic acid; DHA, docosahexaenoic acid; and AA/EPA, ratio. Significant differences in plasma PUFA concentrations were found using analysis of covariance (ANCOVA) analysis after adjustment for age and BMI. Mean ± SD (all such values). $^*P < 0.05$.

Table 2.
*Plasma fatty acid concentrations (μg/mL) for the four groups stratified by the stress level and the presence of PTSD (*n = 563*).*

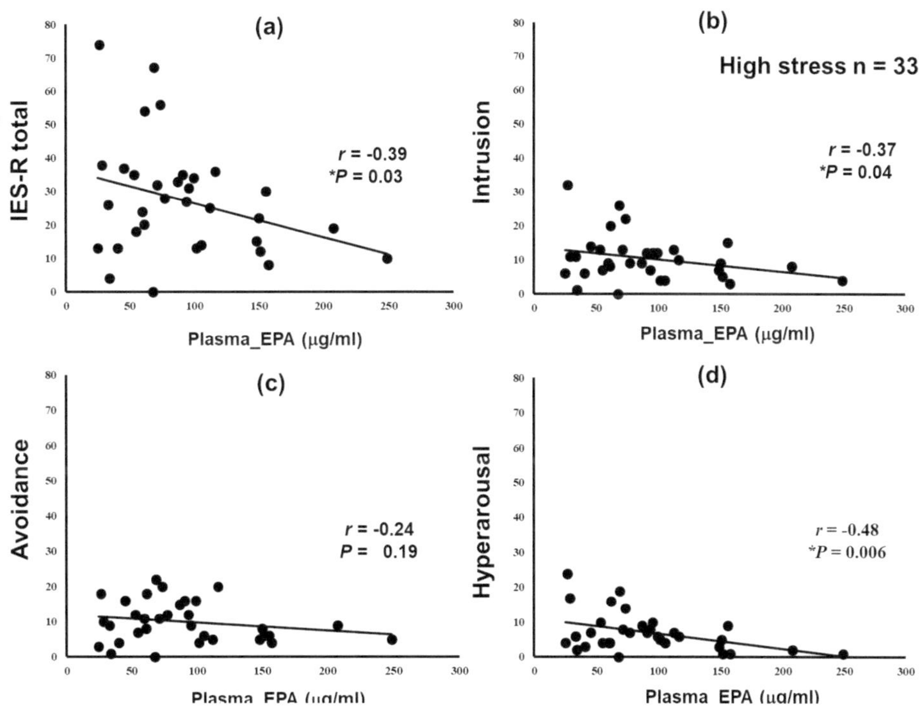

Figure 2.
Scatter plots of plasma EPA level with IES-R scores in the high-stress group. (a) IES-R total, (b) intrusion, (c) avoidance, and (d) hyperarousal. IES-R, impact event scale-revised; r, partial correlation coefficient, controlling for age and BMI.

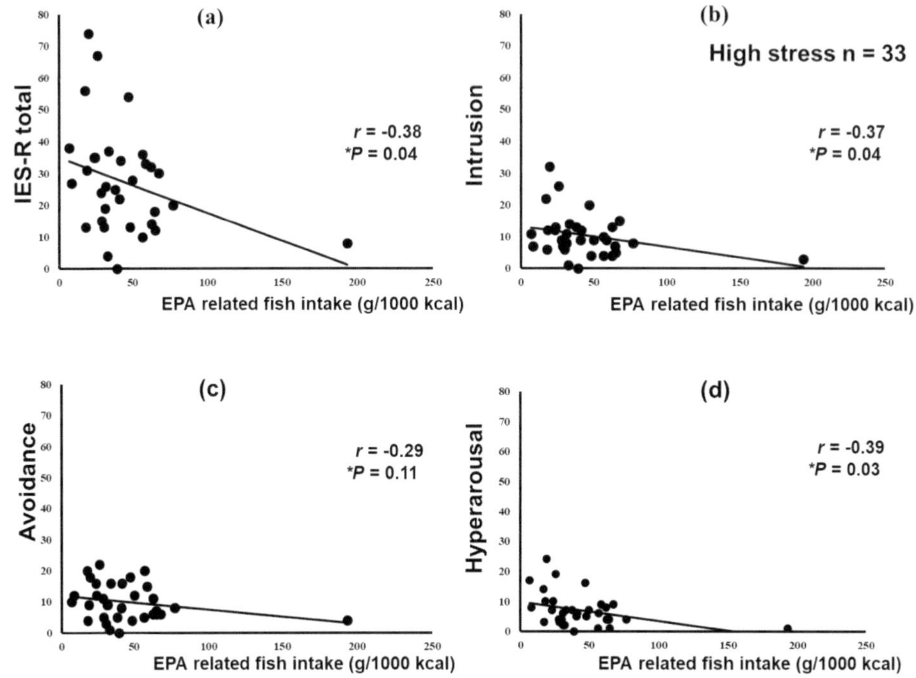

Figure 3.
Scatter plots of EPA-correlated fish intake with IES-R scores in the high-stress group. (a) IES-R total, (b) intrusion, (c) avoidance, and (d) hyperarousal. IES-R, impact event scale-revised; r, partial correlation coefficient, controlling for age and BMI. As shown, there was one individual who had exceptionally high fish intake, which may have biased the results. Even when this individual was excluded, there remained inverse correlations of EPA-correlated fish intake, at least at a trend level, with IES-R total score (r = −0.352, P = 0.057), intrusion (r = −0.343, P = 0.063), and hyperarousal (r = −0.412, P = 0.024), but not with avoidance score (r = −0.224, P = 0.23). EPA-related fish intake (g/1000 kcal): energy adjusted values by density method (g/1000 kcal).

those who had moderate stress. This raises the possibility that higher plasma EPA may have a protective effect on the development of PTSD in the high-stress group.

3.3 Negative correlation between plasma EPA level and PTSD symptoms

Since plasma EPA was found to be associated with PTSD, we then performed the partial correlation analyses between plasma EPA level and IES-R scores, controlling for age and BMI for the high stress and moderate stress groups separately. In the high-stress group, there were significant inverse correlations of plasma EPA level with IES-R total score (r = −0.389, $P = 0.031$), intrusion (r = −0.370, $P = 0.04$), and hyperarousal (r = −0.480, $P = 0.006$), but not with avoidance score (r = −0.240, $P = 0.19$) (**Figure 2**). In the moderate-stress group, however, there was no significant correlation (total score: r = 0.020, $P = 0.64$; intrusion: r = −0.009, $P = 0.84$; avoidance: r = 0.020, $P = 0.65$).

3.4 Association of dietary fish intake and PTSD

Initially, we examined the partial correlation between fish intake and plasma EPA level in the total subjects (N = 563), controlling for age and BMI. Among the six categories of the fish intake (see Section 2), categories 2, 4, 5, and 6 showed a highly significant correlation with plasma EPA (C2: r = 0.127, $P = 0.003$; C4: r = 0.288, $P < 0.001$; C5: r = 0.197, $P < 0.001$; C6: r = 0.158, $P < 0.001$), while categories 1 and 3 did not (both $P > 0.05$). Then, we summed fish intakes of categories 2, 4, 5, and 6 (i.e., C2 + C4 + C5 + C6) to make a variable of "EPA-correlated fish intake." This variable was used for the analysis of the relationship between fish intake and PTSD.

When analyses were performed similarly to plasma EPA, EPA-correlated fish intake tended to be greater in the non-PTSD group than in the PTSD group [$F(1, 29) = 2.99$, $P = 0.094$, partial $\eta^2 = 0.094$] in the high-stress group. Such relationship was not found in the moderate-stress group (data not shown).

Then, we performed partial correlation analyses between EPA-correlated fish intake and IES-R scores. In individuals who experienced high stress, there were significant inverse correlations of EPA-correlated fish intake with IES-R total score (r = −0.377, $P = 0.037$), intrusion (r = −0.370, $P = 0.041$), and hyperarousal (r = −0.393, $P = 0.029$), but not with avoidance score (r = −0.290, $P = 0.11$) (**Figure 3**). In those who had moderate stress, however, there was no significant correlation (data not shown).

4. Discussion

Our main findings can be summarized as follows. Plasma EPA level was higher in the non-PTSD group than in the PTSD group among individuals with high stress but not among those with moderate stress. There was a negative correlation of plasma EPA level with IES-R total, intrusion, and hyperarousal scores in the high stress group. Likewise, EPA-related fish intake showed a negative correlation of plasma EPA level with IES-R total, intrusion, and hyperarousal scores in the high stress group. To our knowledge, this is the first study that elucidated the relationships of plasma EPA as well as fish intake with PTSD in a community sample who suffered from a major natural disaster.

The observed inverse correlations of plasma EPA level with IES-R scores in our study are consistent with the results of Kalinic et al. [11]. Another previous study reported that EPA and AA levels in the serum were both inversely related to the risk for PTSD in subjects of post-motor vehicle accident [10]. However, we did not find such an association for AA. We found no significant correlation of EPA or fish intake with avoidance score. One possible reason for this lack of correlation might be that our subjects were recruited from those who remained to be living in the disaster area and thus people who could not live the area because of avoidance had not been enrolled in the study.

Although the cross-sectional nature of the study precludes to determine the causal relationship, our findings raise the possibility that dietary intake or supplement to increase EPA level has a protective effect on the development of PTSD in severely stressed people. In line, there is some evidence that increase in EPA reduces the risk of PTSD. Matsuoka et al. examined the effect of DHA/EPA capsules (1 capsule: 320 mg of oil with 70% DHA and 7% EPA, 7 capsules/day) on the development of PTSD among Japanese disaster medical assistance team members after the Great East Japan Earthquake and Tsunami [6]. The DHA/EPA capsules were found to only slightly reduce PTSD symptoms among female members; however, it had no effect among male members, suggesting that DHA has no major benefit in the prevention of PTSD. However, subsequent secondary analyses revealed that elevation in erythrocyte EPA levels after the supplementation seem to be effective in alleviation of PTSD symptoms and QOL [8, 9]. These findings are consistent with our findings that plasma EPA, but not DHA, was associated with PTSD.

In our analyses, plasma EPA level was highly positively correlated with fish intake of categories 2, 4, 5, and 6, that is, whole-eat fish, dried fish/salted fish, oil-rich fish, and non-oil-rich fish. This means that eating habits are strongly reflected in plasma EPA, and taking EPA-correlated fishes may have a beneficial effect. Notably, the Great East Japan Earthquake and Tsunami caused the Fukushima nuclear power plant accident. The release of radioactive water from the nuclear power station had a negative impact upon fish consumption in the adjacent areas, including Kitaibaraki city, which may have further increased the risk of PTSD.

Accumulating evidence has suggested that inflammation plays an important role in the pathogenesis of PTSD [3]. The meta-analysis of 20 studies revealed that PTSD is associated with increased interleukin 6, interleukin 1β, TNFα, and interferon γ levels, suggesting chronic low-grade inflammation as a potential target or biomarker in PTSD treatment [20]. Recently, our group obtained further evidence for increased IL-6 in female PTSD patients, most of whom developed the illness after domestic violence, compared with controls [21]. EPA together with DHA are capable of inhibiting many aspects of inflammation including leucocyte chemotaxis, adhesion molecule expression and leucocyte-endothelial adhesive interactions, production of eicosanoids like prostaglandins and leukotrienes from the n-6 fatty acid arachidonic acid, and production of pro-inflammatory cytokines [22]. Local-acting lipid mediators termed resolvins and protectins generated from EPA and DHA have also been known to resolve inflammation and protect the tissue [23]. EPA and DHA offer different benefits, and the suppressive effect of EPA on cytokine production seems to be more pronounced as compared to DHA [24]. EPA is rapidly oxidized in the brain, and thus, it has a short lifespan [25]. Therefore, the brain may need a constant supply of EPA to inhibit neuroinflammation.

This study had several limitations. First, we used non-fasting blood samples for PUFA measurement. However, it has been suggested that fasting is largely unnecessary for routine lipid level determinations [26]. Indeed, plasma EPA level well correlated with recent fish intake (i.e., C2, C4, C5, C6) in our subjects. Second, we assessed PTSD symptoms by using the IES-R questionnaire rather than a structured interview by clinicians (e.g., clinician-administered PTSD scale by Blake et al. [27]). Third, the assessment of food intake was also performed by self-report brief questionnaire (BDHQ). Finally, the sample size was small, particularly for the subjects who experienced high stress (N = 33). Further studies in a larger sample size will be required to draw more robust results.

5. Conclusion

We examined the association of plasma PUFA levels and dietary fish intake with the development of PTSD in a population-based sample of 563 women struck by the Great East Japan Earthquake and Tsunami. Plasma EPA level was higher in the non-PTSD group than in the PTSD group among individuals with high stress but not among those with moderate stress. There was a negative correlation of plasma EPA level with IES-R total, intrusion, and hyperarousal scores in the high stress group. Similarly, EPA-related fish intake showed a negative correlation of plasma EPA level with IES-R total, intrusion, and hyperarousal scores in the high stress group. Taken together, higher plasma EPA level and EPA-increasing fish intake are associated with lower risk for PTSD in individuals who have experienced severe stress in a natural disaster. Our findings provide support for the use of nutritional intervention in preventing and alleviating PTSD.

Acknowledgements

We thank all of the participants in this study and the staff of Kitaibaraki Restoration Project who collected the epidemiological data and blood sample. The responsibilities of the authors were as follows: E.A.: Data analysis, interpretation of study findings, and manuscript writing. M.O. and K.H.: Supervision of data collection and data analysis. I.I. & N.K.: Preparation of the study and data collection.

S.S. & T.A.: Conception and design of the study. H.K.: Conception and design of the study, supervision of the study, and manuscript writing. This study was supported by a Health and Labor Sciences Research Grant for Comprehensive Research on Persons with Disabilities (T.A. & H.K.).

Conflict of interest

None of the authors have any conflicts of interest.

Abbreviations

AA	arachidonic acid
ANOVA	analysis of variance
BDHQ	brief-type self-administered diet history questionnaire
DHA	docosahexaenoic acid
EPA	eicosapentaenoic acid
IES-R	impact event scale-revised
MANCOVA	multiple analysis of covariance
PTSD	posttraumatic stress disorder
PUFA	polyunsaturated fatty acid

Author details

Emiko Aizawa[1,2], Miho Ota[1,3], Ikki Ishida[1], Norie Koga[1], Kotaro Hattori[1,4], Shinji Sato[3,5], Takashi Asada[3,6] and Hiroshi Kunugi[1*]

1 Department of Mental Disorder Research, National Institute of Neuroscience, National Center of Neurology and Psychiatry, Tokyo, Japan

2 Department of Human Life Science, Nagoya University of Economics, Aichi, Japan

3 Department of Neuropsychiatry, University of Tsukuba, Ibaraki, Japan

4 Department of Bioresources, Medical Genome Center, National Institute of Neuroscience, National Center of Neurology and Psychiatry, Tokyo, Japan

5 Department of Psychiatry, Ibaraki Clinical Educational and Training Center, Faculty of Medicine, University of Tsukuba, Ibaraki, Japan

6 Center for Brain Integration Research, Tokyo Medical and Dental University, Tokyo, Japan

*Address all correspondence to: hkunugi@ncnp.go.jp

References

[1] Javidi H, Yadollahie M. Post-traumatic stress disorder. Indian Journal of Occupational and Environmental Medicine. 2012;**3**:2-9

[2] Wilson CB, McLaughlin LD, Nair A, Ebenezer PJ, Dange R, Francis J. Inflammation and oxidative stress are elevated in the brain, blood, and adrenal glands during the progression of post-traumatic stress disorder in a predator exposure animal model. PLoS One. 2013;**8**:e76146

[3] Hori H, Kim Y. Inflammation and post-traumatic stress disorder. Psychiatry and Clinical Neurosciences. 2019;**73**:143-153. DOI: 10.1111/pcn.12820

[4] Watts BV, Schnurr PP, Mayo L, Young-Xu Y, Weeks WB, Friedman MJ. Meta-analysis of the efficacy of treatments for posttraumatic stress disorder. The Journal of Clinical Psychiatry. 2013;**74**:e541-e550

[5] Hashimoto M, Maekawa M, Katakura M, Hamazaki K, Matsuoka Y. Possibility of polyunsaturated fatty acids for the prevention and treatment of neuropsychiatric illnesses. Journal of Pharmacological Sciences. 2014;**124**:294-300

[6] Matsuoka Y, Nishi D, Nakaya N, Sone T, Hamazaki K, Hamazaki T, et al. Attenuating posttraumatic distress with omega-3 polyunsaturated fatty acids among disaster medical assistance team members after the Great East Japan Earthquake: The APOP randomized controlled trial. BMC Psychiatry. 2011;**11**:132

[7] Matsuoka Y, Nishi D, Hamazaki K, Yonemoto N, Matsumura K, Noguchi H, et al. Docosahexaenoic acid for selective prevention of posttraumatic stress disorder among severely injured patients: A randomized, placebo-controlled trial. The Journal of Clinical Psychiatry. 2015;**76**:e1015-e1022

[8] Matsuoka YJ, Hamazaki K, Nishi D, Hamazaki T. Change in blood levels of eicosapentaenoic acid and posttraumatic stress symptom: A secondary analysis of data from a placebo-controlled trial of omega3 supplements. Journal of Affective Disorders. 2016;**205**:289-291

[9] Noguchi H, Nishi D, Matsumura K, Hamazaki K, Hamazaki T, Matsuoka YJ. Limited effect of omega-3 fatty acids on the quality of life in survivors of traumatic injury: A randomized, placebo-controlled trial. Prostaglandins, Leukotrienes, and Essential Fatty Acids. 2017;**127**:1-5

[10] Matsuoka Y, Nishi D, Hamazaki K. Serum levels of polyunsaturated fatty acids and the risk of posttraumatic stress disorder. Psychotherapy and Psychosomatics. 2013;**82**:408-410

[11] Kalinic D, Borovac Stefanovic L, Jeroncic A, Mimica N, Dodig G, Delas I. Eicosapentaenoic acid in serum lipids could be inversely correlated with severity of clinical symptomatology in Croatian war veterans with posttraumatic stress disorder. Croatian Medical Journal. 2014;**55**:27-37

[12] Gill JM, Szanton SL, Page GG. Biological underpinnings of health alterations in women with PTSD: A sex disparity. Biological Research for Nursing. 2005;7:44-54

[13] World Medical Assocition. World medical association declaration of Helsinki: Ethical principles for medical reseach involving humansubjects. JAMA. 2000;**284**:3043-3045

[14] Asukai N, Kato H, Kawamura N, et al. Reliability and validity of the Japanese-language version of the impact of event scale-revised (IES-R-J): Four

studies of different traumatic events. The Journal of Nervous and Mental Disease. 2002;**190**:175-182

[15] Horowitz M, Wilner N, Alvarez W. Impact of event scale: A measure of subjective stress. Psychosomatic Medicine. 1979;**41**:209-218

[16] Numata T, Gunfan S, Takayama S, Takahashi S, Monma Y, Kaneko S, et al. Treatment of posttraumatic stress disorder using the traditional Japanese herbal medicine saikokeishikankyoto: A randomized, observer-blinded, controlled trial in survivors of the Great East Japan Earthquake and Tsunami. Evidence-based Complementary and Alternative Medicine. 2014;**2014**:683293

[17] Sasaki S, Yanagibori R, Amano K. Self-administered diet history questionnaire developed for health education: A relative validation of the test-version by comparison with 3-day diet record in women. Journal of Epidemiology. 1998;**8**:203-215

[18] Kobayashi S, Murakami K, Sasaki S, Okubo H, Hirota N, Notsu A, et al. Comparison of relative validity of food group intakes estimated by comprehensive and brief-type self-administered diet history questionnaires against 16 d dietary records in Japanese adults. Public Health Nutrition. 2011;**14**:1200-1211

[19] Takemoto Y, Suzuki Y, Horibe R, Shimozawa N, Wanders RJ, Kondo N. Gas chromatography/mass spectrometry analysis of very long chain fatty acids, docosahexaenoic acid, phytanic acid and plasmalogen for the screening of peroxisomal disorders. Brain and Development. 2003;**25**:481-487

[20] Passos IC, Vasconcelos-Moreno MP, Costa LG, et al. Inflammatory markers in post-traumatic stress disorder: A systematic review, meta-analysis, and meta-regression. Lancet Psychiatry. 2015;**2**:1002-1012

[21] Imai R, Hori H, Itoh M, Lin M, Niwa M, Ino K, et al. Inflammatory markers and their possible effects on cognitive function in women with posttraumatic stress disorder. Journal of Psychiatric Research. 2018;**102**:192-200

[22] Calder PC. Marine omega-3 fatty acids and inflammatory processes: Effects, mechanisms and clinical relevance. Biochimica et Biophysica Acta. 2015;**1851**:469-484

[23] Serhan CN, Yacoubian S, Yang R. Anti-inflammatory and proresolving lipid mediators. Annual Review of Pathology. 2008;**3**:279-312

[24] Gorjao R, Azevedo-Martins AK, Rodrigues HG, Abdulkader F, Arcisio-Miranda M, Procopio J, et al. Comparative effects of DHA and EPA on cell function. Pharmacology & Therapeutics. 2009;**122**:56-64

[25] Chen CT, Liu Z, Bazinet RP. Rapid de-esterification and loss of eicosapentaenoic acid from rat brain phospholipids: An intracerebroventricular study. Journal of Neurochemistry. 2011;**116**:363-373

[26] Sidhu D, Naugler C. Fasting time and lipid levels in a community-based population: A cross-sectional study. Archives of Internal Medicine. 2012;**172**:1707-1710

[27] Blake DD, Weathers FW, Nagy LM, Kaloupek DG, Gusman FD, Charney DS, et al. The development of a clinician-administered PTSD scale. Journal of Traumatic Stress. 1995;**8**:75-90

Chapter 4

Borderline Personality Disorder and Childhood Trauma: The Posited Mechanisms of Symptoms Expression

Maria Uscinska, Nicolo' Gagliano, Andrea Polla Mattiot and Silvio Bellino

Abstract

Traumatic events are reported in a large percentage of the population, however, only in some individuals it will lead to a diagnosable trauma-related disorder. Borderline personality disorder (BPD) is deemed to be a form of acute reaction to childhood trauma. Therein experiences of childhood abuse and neglect take on an important etiological role, generating severely disorganized attachment relationships, which in turn affect the development of emotional regulation systems, and significantly inhibit the development of mentalization and metacognitive skills. Furthermore, the last decade has seen important contribution of neuroscientific research in shedding light on the neurobiological correlates of traumatic experiences. A wealth of scientific literature links the onset of BPD to the combination between genetic and environmental factors (G×E), in particular between biological vulnerabilities and the exposure to traumatic experiences during childhood. Although no research can predict with certainty which trauma will translate into symptoms, there are indications as to who is more at risk of developing a trauma-related disorder. Herein we describe the psychological and epigenetic mechanisms affected by childhood trauma and altered in BPD patients.

Keywords: borderline personality disorder, childhood trauma, psychopathology

1. Historical and conceptual overview

The concept of trauma first entered the DSM-III as a rare, catastrophic stressor outside the range of usual human experience, apt to evoke significant symptoms of distress in most people [1]. To date, it is deemed a silent epidemic [2] defined in DSM-5 as a result of either direct or indirect exposure to actual or threatened serious injury or sexual violence, death or a threatened death [3]. Meaning 'stroke or wound' in Greek, in psychopathology trauma refers to a lesion or an insult to the psychic organism induced by a stressor or a series of noxious events that occur suddenly and in a disruptive way in a subject's life [4].

The impact of trauma on the human psyche has received considerable research attention, starting with the thesis that it is a process taking place within the attachment relationships and separation [5]. Owing to the advent of neuroimaging techniques it is well-established that human experiences, whether traumatic or therapeutic, have

IntechOpen

measurable influences on the brain structure and function. As harmful pathways are etched deep into the brain following an exposure to trauma, neuroimaging studies allow to index the extend of associated cerebral damage. Therein, the level of maternal support in childhood was shown to determine hippocampus volume in adulthood [6], whilst childhood poverty was associated with reduced white matter, cortical gray matter, and hippocampal volume [7]. In some cases, the progressive impact of traumatic experience may lead to a diagnosis of debilitating psychiatric disorders such as BPD, complex PTSD or disorders of extreme stress, not otherwise specified (DESNOS) [8]. A wealth of research on neuro-functional alterations associated with trauma-exposure revealed patterns of increased amygdala activity in response to threatening stimuli, and simultaneous decreased activity in prefrontal areas of the cortex that downregulates the amygdala [9–11], as well as hyperactive hippocampus [11]. Furthermore, recent evidence has shown that trauma experience is associated with altered functional connectivity between the amygdala, and medial prefrontal cortex (mPFC), insula, and dCCA [10, 12], furthering the thesis of an interplay between prefrontal regions and limbic structures. With this in mind, the next section follows with an overview of trauma-related psychiatric disorders. In keeping with research trends in developmental neurosciences the main theme of the chapter is pathological pathways from trauma to BPD, focusing on trauma-induced alterations in neurobiological systems.

2. The interface between trauma and mental illness

Mental illness is often broadly defined, encompassing disturbances across domains of functioning in the emotional, cognitive, and/or behavioral realms. Accordingly, the biopsychosocial model of disease causation and treatment brought about a new way of conceptualizing mental health difficulties resulting from biological, psychological, and social factors [13]. In this view, adverse life events interact with genetic susceptibility, personality and social context to co-determine individual vulnerability to clinical expression of mental illness, its severity and course. In quest to unravel how different factors and processes translate into a psychiatric disturbance, researchers and clinicians have sought to understand the progressive and developmental impact of trauma experience on an individual. A wealth of research reveals that exposure to adversities, stressors and neglect can chronically and pervasively alter biological, cognitive, psychological, and social development, giving rise to disturbances in impulse and affect regulation, alterations in attention, consciousness, attribution and schema, as well as interpersonal difficulties [14–16]. On the neurobiological level, exposure to trauma triggers a surge of neurochemical factors, potent enough to interfere with integrative capacity and the ordinary process of neurodevelopment [17, 18]. Therein appraisal of adverse events and associated emotions might give rise to the stress response, prompting a cascade of biological events that alter various essential processes, namely neurogenesis, synaptogenesis, migration and neurochemical differentiation. Indeed, research exists to support that a persistent traumatic event might induce a permanent neurobiological modification of the subject's stress response [19] evidenced in elevated urinary epinephrine, norepinephrine, and dopamine, increase or decrease in baseline heart rate, alterations of alpha-2-adrenergic receptors, limbic and cortical abnormalities, and altered development of some cortical areas [18]. Elevated stress in turn has been shown to downregulate the process of hippocampal neurogenesis [20]. Notably, peritraumatic stress reactions within the first hours are predictors of the development of a trauma-related disorder, and therefore constitute a critical window for interventions for prevention of trauma-related disorders [21, 22]. This is presumably due to the fact that memory consolidation occurs during the first night's sleep following the exposure [23]. Conversely, it has been shown that an adequate resilience capacity, that is the ability to adapt to an adverse situation is a crucial protective factor against the occurrence of a trauma-related disorder [24].

3. Trauma-related disorders in DSM-5

Unlike previous editions, DSM-5 has introduced a number of modifications, regrouping disorders that appear to be etiologically related to one another [3]. In this view, trauma- and stress-related disorders are separated from anxiety disorders and obsessive–compulsive disorder, and classified in a specific chapter clustering disorders characterized by the occurrence of one or more traumatic or stressful events in which the subject is involved. The cluster includes Post-Traumatic Stress Disorder (PTSD), Acute Stress Disorder (ASD), Attachment Disorders, Disinhibited Social Engagement Disorder (DSED) and Adjustment Disorder. Whilst Attachment Disorders and DSED originate in childhood, the remaining diagnoses refer to trauma experience in the adult population [3].

PTSD is the most complex disturbance of the cluster, characterized by intrusive re-experiencing symptoms and avoidant, numbing, and hyperarousal symptoms that manifest themselves after an insult to the person's physical integrity or event that has caused a serious injury to the subject or to the other close to him/her [3, 18]. Unlike previous versions, DSM-5 lists specific criteria of PTSD symptoms for patients under 6 years of age, which may not be particularly manifest or verbally expressed, nevertheless a careful observation of the child's behavior can identify the impact of trauma on interpersonal difficulties, insecure disorganized attachment style, or episodes of aggression and difficulty in affective regulation [25].

ASD encompasses a broad array of immediate, transient reactions to a sudden impact of trauma that typically subsides within 48 hours. The disorder is characterized by intrusive memories, negative mood, dissociation, avoidance, and/or hyperarousal experienced during the first month after a traumatic event. Since the introduction of ASD into DSM-IV in order to identify those at risk for developing PTSD, concerns have been raised whether the diagnosis reliably predicted PTSD and whether it pathologized normal reactions to trauma. Furthermore, little empirical evidence exists to support the thesis that an individual with ASD endorses at least three dissociative symptoms. In response to this criticism, the ASD diagnostic criteria were changed with the publication of DSM-5 excluding the dissociative symptoms requirement resulting in a stronger predictive power.

Adjustment disorder has been described as the linchpin between normalcy and psychiatric disturbance as it characterizes a severe emotional reaction to an identifiable stressor that does not meet criteria for other more specific disorder [26]. The symptoms can vary among diagnosed individuals and include hopelessness, anhedonia, sadness, irritability, sleep problems, avoidance, diminished performance, aggression and so forth.

Attachment disorders are characterized by a disrupted attachment related to early social deprivation, maltreatment or neglect and are differentiated into disinhibited and inhibited or reactive attachment disorders. Whilst the former is associated with the absence of early attachment relationships and indiscriminate sociability, the latter is etiologically linked to neglect and abuse.

4. Trauma and borderline personality disorder

The interface between childhood trauma and Borderline Personality Disorder (BPD) has been a topic of discussion and controversy in clinical research. This

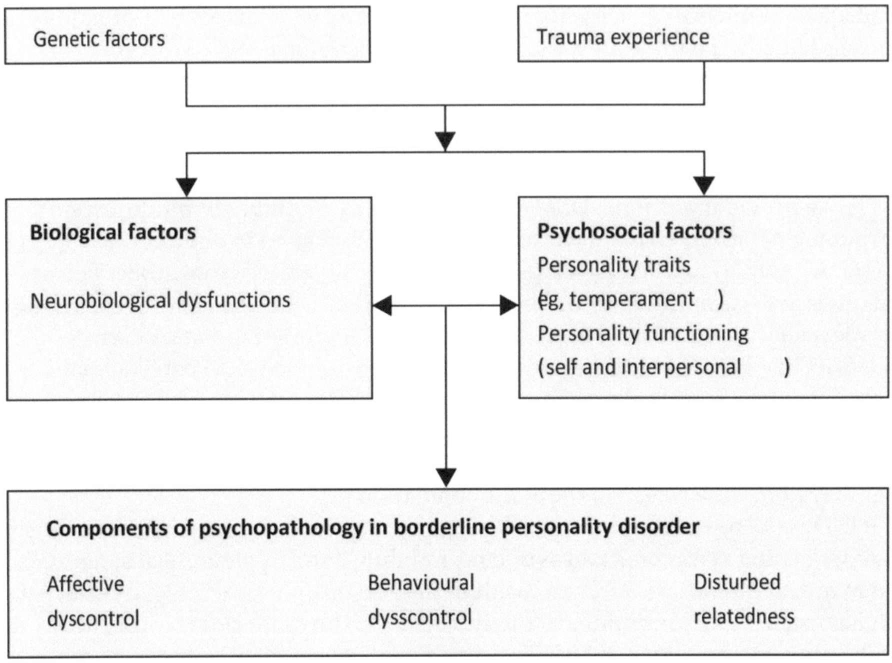

Figure 1.
The biopsychosocial model of borderline personality disorder.

severe psychiatric disorder is characterized by a pervasive pattern of instability in affect regulation, impulse control, self-image, cognition and interpersonal relationships [3]. Frequent self-damaging and impulsive behaviors, such as suicide, self-harm or substance abuse exacerbate the severity and morbidity of the disorder [27, 28]. Although the diagnosis of BPD does not require a history of traumatic event, childhood trauma is considered the main environmental factor contributing to the etiology and severity of the disorder [29–31]. By way of example, in a prospective study 500 children who had suffered physical and sexual abuse and neglect were found to be significantly more likely to meet criteria for BPD in adulthood than matched controls [32]. Although childhood trauma does not always lead to psychopathology [31] there is an empirical consensus that the interaction between childhood trauma and temperamental traits constitutes the basis for the etiology and severity of BPD [33, 34]. Accordingly, the biopsychosocial model of BPD (**Figure 1**) posits that the disorder results from the interaction between biologically based temperamental vulnerabilities and adverse experiences in childhood [35–38].

5. Clinical pathways from trauma to BPD

5.1 Psychodynamic psychopathology and attachment

From the standpoint of contemporary clinical psychology there are three perspectives firmly rooted in the attachment theory that best describe the complex psychopathology of BPD, namely the processes of mentalization, the theory of interpersonal motivational systems and the model of affective regulation.

5.1.1 Mentalization

A trauma within the bond of attachment goes to generate a repeated and continuous activation of this system. Whilst looking for closeness of an attachment figure that has been traumatizing, the child will reencounter traumatic experiences. The prolonged activation of the attachment system will produce specific inhibitory responses to the mentalization, as well as those related to the physiological increase of emotional arousal. The child, in an attempt to obtain some form of control over the aggressor, might try to identify with the aggressor, internalizing the intent of the aggressor and thus generating a part of the dissociated self, so-called the alien Self.

Over time, the destructive intent of the abuser will be perceived as coming from within own self and not from another person, leading to experimenting a strong sense of hatred towards oneself by child that might persist to adulthood. To deal with severe trauma and abuse a defensive operation to avoid the reflection on the content of the caregiver's mind is triggered, thereby preventing the resolution of the experiences of abuse [39].

This mechanism explains why BPD patients frequently have relationships in which they feel victimized by others perceived as persecutors. Through the defensive process called projective identification, a patient might attempt to "force" a significant person, including the psychotherapist, to assume the character of the "Alien Self/Bad Object".

5.1.2 Attachment and other interpersonal motivational systems

In accordance with the theory of attachment, the experience of ill-treatment in the evolutionary age can have a strong negative impact on the development of the models of representation of the Self, of the figures of attachment and of the relationship between them.

The theory of interpersonal motivational systems [40–42] identifies a series of systems similar to that of attachment, which are also evolutionary-based, and support individuals towards some fundamental goals of existence such as defense, attachment, care, social rank, sexuality, cooperation, predation. According to Liotti, the disorganization of attachment involves both a multifaceted and split representation of oneself and the figure of attachment, and a metaphysical deficit that makes affective regulation difficult. The structuring of an internal disorganized operating model with perceptions of the multiple self-object relationship, inconsistent and not integrated, it seems explainable through the simultaneous and incompatible activation of the attachment and defense system in the child, as the caregiver deputed to respond to the demands of the attachment system is also the figure activating the defense system endangering the child's personal life and safety. Once they reach adulthood, when traumatic memories emerge in the mind of the parents, the pain associated with them activates the attachment system of the figures that should provide care, thus evoking feelings of anger and fear in the caregiver when care responses are needed by the baby.

5.1.3 Affective regulation

The theory of affective regulation [43–47] focuses more on the psychobiological or "primary" aspects of the affective experience rather than cognitive-affective aspects of the experience as indicated in the work of Fonagy and colleagues.

Incorporating contributions of the clinical tradition of psychology of the Self [48] and contemporary infant research [49, 50], the theory proposes the process of tuning, defined as the synchronicity of affective states as the foundation of caregiving practices and the most compromised aspect in the relationships of attachment. Failure to tune between the child's affective states and the caregiver prevents the affective adjustment process within the 'tolerance window' which constitutes the ideal metabolic conditions for neuronal metabolic development.

5.2 Cognitive psychopathology

Beck and collaborators [51] have provided a conceptualization of the BPD according to the cognitive-behavioral perspective, which posits three main dysfunctional nuclear convictions at the basis if the disorder, namely the world is dangerous and malicious, I am powerless and vulnerable, and I am inherently unacceptable. The first two convictions tend to produce a sense of hypervigilance and distrust of others. There are two other central cognitive features: a dichotomic thought and a poorly articulated self-pattern, which determine a weak sense of personal identity. These aspects contribute to creating the emotional and interpersonal behaviors typical of this disorder.

Within the schema therapy framework Young and colleagues [52] stress that borderline subjects tend to present too many schemas and to oscillate between extreme affective states, and it is in the excess and overlap of reference schemas that the symptomatology of the BPD resides.

Dialectical Behavior Therapy (DBT) posits at the center of the borderline disorder a deficit of the system of regulation of the emotions with its consequences among which are: understanding the contextual, relational and transient nature of emotions; building an effective mental model of the relationships between emotions and environmental events; and semantically labeling each emotion properly [53]. This deficit is deemed to be the product of temperamental characteristics, such as emotional vulnerability, which interact with a disabling environment of the person's emotional experiences.

According to the cognitive constructivist model proposed by Dimaggio and Semerari [54] BPD is attributable to specific functional deficits of metacognition capabilities, detectable in the following functions:

- deficit of integration, where different mental states are experimented without reciprocal memory (hence, the tendency to oscillate between them in little chaotic and rapid modulated);

- deficit in emotional regulation, caused by a genetic-temperamental vulnerability that results in hyperreactivity to stimuli, combined with environmental-disabling experiences;

- deficit of differentiation between reality and its representations as a consequence of affective dysregulation.

The relationship between these deficits is manifold, where dysregulation and integration difficulties affect each other, leading to a lack of differentiation.

Conflict of interest

The author has no relevant affiliations or financial involvement with any organization or entity with a financial interest in or financial conflict with the subject matter or materials discussed in the manuscript. This includes employment, consultancies, honoraria, stock ownership or options, expert testimony, grants or patents received or pending, or royalties. No writing assistance was utilized in the production of this manuscript.

Author details

Maria Uscinska[1*], Nicolo' Gagliano[2], Andrea Polla Mattiot[3] and Silvio Bellino[3]

1 Centre for Personality Disorders, Department of Neurosciences, University of Turin, Italy

2 Radiodiagnostics, Radiotherapy and Nuclear Medicine, Humanitas Research Hospital, Milan, Italy

3 Centre for Personality Disorders, Molinette Hospital, Turin, Italy

*Address all correspondence to: maria.uscinska@edu.unito.it

References

[1] American Psychiatric Association. Diagnostic and Statistical Manual of Mental Disorders. 3rd ed. Washington, DC: American Psychiatric Association; 1980

[2] Kaffman A. The silent epidemic of neurodevelopmental injuries. Biological Psychiatry. 2009;**66**(7):624-626. DOI: 10.1016/j.biopsych.2009.08.002

[3] American Psychiatric Association. Diagnostic and Statistical Manual of Mental Disorders. 5th ed. Washington, DC: American Psychiatric Association; 2013

[4] Siracusano A. Manuale di Psichiatria. Rome: II pensiero scientifico; 2014

[5] Bowlby J. Attachment and Loss. New York: Basic; 1969

[6] Luby J, Barch DM, Belden A, Gaffrey MS, Tillman R, Babb C, et al. Maternal support in early childhood predicts larger hippocampal volumes at school age. Proceedings of the National Academy of Sciences of the United States of America. 2012;**109**(8):2854-2859. DOI: 10.1073/pnas.1118003109

[7] Luby J, Belden A, Botteron K, Marrus N, Harms MP, Babb C, et al. The effects of poverty on childhood brain development: The mediating effect of caregiving and stressful life events. Journal of American Medical Association Pediatrics. 2013;**167**(12):1135-1142. DOI: 10.1001/jamapediatrics.2013.3139

[8] Cattane N, Rossi R, Landfredi M, Cattaneo A. Borderline personality disorder and childhood trauma: Exploring the affected biological systems and mechanisms. BMC Psychiatry. 2017;**17**:221. DOI: 10.1186/s12888-017-1383-2

[9] Rauch SL, Shin LM, Phelps EA. Neurocircuitry models of posttraumatic stress disorder and extinction: Human neuroimaging research—Past, present, and future. Biological Psychiatry. 2006;**60**:376-382. DOI: 10.1016/j.biopsych.2006.06.004

[10] Hayes JP, Hayes SM, Mikedis AM. Quantitative meta-analysis of neural activity in posttraumatic stress disorder. Biology of Mood & Anxiety Disorders. 2012;**2**:9. DOI: 10.1186/2045-5380-2-9

[11] Patel R, Spreng RN, Shin LM, Girard TA. Neurocircuitry models of posttraumatic stress disorder and beyond: A meta-analysis of functional neuroimaging studies. Neuroscience and Biobehavioral Reviews. 2012;**36**:2130-2142. DOI: 10.1016/j.neubiorev.2012.06.003

[12] Stevens JS, Jovanovic T, Fani N, Ely TD, Glover EM, Bradley B. Disrupted amygdala-prefrontal functional connectivity in civilian women with posttraumatic stress disorder. Journal of Psychiatric Research. 2013;**47**:1469-1478. DOI: 10.1016/j.jpsychires.2013.05.031

[13] Engel GL. The need for a new medical model: A challenge for biomedicine. Science. 1977;**196**:129-136. Available from: http://www.jstor.org/stable/1743658

[14] Burns BJ, Hoagwood K, Maultsby LT, Epstein MH, Kutash K, Duchnowski A. Improving outcomes for children and adolescents with serious emotional and behavioral disorders: Current and future directions. In: Epstein M, Kutash K, Duchnowski A, editors. Outcomes for Children and Youth with Emotional and Behavioral Disorders and Their Families: Programs and Evaluation Best Practices. Austin, TX: PRO-ED; 1998. pp. 685-707

[15] Cook A, Spinazzola J, Ford J, Lanktree C, Blaustein M, Cloitre M,

et al. Complex trauma in children and adolescents. Psychiatric Annals. 2005;**35**:390-398. DOI: 10.3928/00485713-20050501-05

[16] Spinazzola J, Ford JD, Zucker M, van der Kolk BA, Silva S, Smith SF, et al. Survey evaluates complex trauma exposure, outcome, and intervention among children and adolescents. Psychiatric Annals. 2005;**35**:433-439

[17] Gonzalez A, Del Rio-Casanova L, Justo-Alonso A. Integrating neurobiology of emotion regulation and trauma therapy: Reflections on EMDR therapy. Reviews in the Neurosciences. 2017;**28**(4):431-440. DOI: 10.1515/revneuro-2016-0070

[18] Yehuda R, Hoge CW, McFarlane AC, Vermetten E, Lanius RA, Nievergelt CM, et al. Posttraumatic stress disorder. Nature Reviews. Disease Primers. 2015;**1**:15057. DOI: 10.1038/nrdp.2015.57

[19] Jeter WK, Brannon LA. Moving beyond "sticks and stones": Chronic psychological trauma predicts posttraumatic stress symptoms. Journal of Trauma & Dissociation. 2014;**15**(5):548-556. DOI: 10.1080/15299732.2014.907596

[20] Gould E, Tanapat P. Stress and hippocampal neurogenesis. Biological Psychiatry. 1999;**46**(11):1472-1479

[21] Moller A, Sondergaard HP, Helstrom L. Tonic immobility during sexual assault—A common reaction predicting post-traumatic stress disorder and severe depression. Acta Obstetricia et Gynecologica Scandinavica. 2017;**96**(8):932-938. DOI: 10.1111/aogs.13174

[22] Gandubert C, Scali J, Ancelin ML, Carriere I, Dupuy AM, Bagnolini G, et al. Biological and psychological predictors of posttraumatic stress disorder onset and chronicity. A one-year prospective study. Neurobiology of Stress. 2016;**3**:61-67. DOI: 10.1016/j.ynstr.2016.02.002

[23] Birmes P, Brunet A, Carreras D, Ducasse JL, Charlet JP, Lauque D, et al. The predictive power of peritraumatic dissociation and acute stress symptoms for posttraumatic stress symptoms: A three-month prospective study. The American Journal of Psychiatry. 2003;**160**(7):1337-1339. DOI: 10.1176/appi.ajp.160.7.1337

[24] Bonanno GA. Loss, trauma, and human resilience: Have we underestimated the human capacity to thrive after extremely aversive events? The American Psychologist. 2004;**59**(1):20-28. DOI: 10.1037/0003-066X.59.1.20

[25] Perrin S. Children exposed to trauma should be screened for symptoms of PTSD. Evidence-Based Mental Health. 2014;**17**(4):107. DOI: 10.1136/eb-2014-101888

[26] Strain JJ, Diefenbacher A. The adjustment disorders: The conundrums of the diagnoses. Comprehensive Psychiatry. 2008;**49**:121-130. DOI: 10.1016/ j.comppsych

[27] Lieb K, Zanarini MC, Schmahl C, Linehan MM, Bohus M. Borderline personality disorder. Lancet. 2004;**364**(9432):453-461

[28] Soloff PH, Lis JA, Kelly T, Cornelius J, Ulrich R. Risk factors for suicidal behaviour in borderline personality disorder. The American Journal of Psychiatry. 1994;**151**(9):1316-1323

[29] Johnson JG, Cohen P, Brown J, Smailes EM, Bernstein DP. Childhood maltreatment increases risk for personality disorders during early adulthood. Archives of General Psychiatry. 1999;**56**:600-606

[30] Johnson JG, Cohen P, Smailes EM, Skodol AE, Brown J, Oldham JM.

Childhood verbal abuse and risk for personality disorders during adolescence and early adulthood. Comprehensive Psychiatry. 2001;**42**:16-23

[31] Spataro J, Mullen PE, Burgess PM, Wells DL, Moss SA. Impact of child sexual abuse on mental health: Prospective study in males and females. The British Journal of Psychiatry. 2004;**184**:416-421

[32] Widom CS, Czaja SJ, Paris J. A prospective investigation of borderline personality disorder in abused and neglected children followed up into adulthood. Journal of Personality Disorders. 2009;**23**:433-446

[33] Laporte L, Paris J, Guttman H, Russell J. Psychopathology, childhood trauma, and personality traits in patients with borderline personality disorder and their sisters. Journal of Personality Disorders. 2011;**25**:448-462

[34] Gratz KL, Latzman RD, Tull MT, Reynolds EK, Lejuez CW. Exploring the association between emotional abuse and childhood borderline personality features: The moderating role of personality traits. Behavior Therapy. 2011;**42**:493-508

[35] Linehan MM. Cognitive-Behavioral Treatment for Borderline Personality Disorder. New York: The Guilford Press; 1993

[36] Zanarini MC, Frankenburg FR. Pathways to the development of borderline personality disorder. Journal of Personality Disorders. 1997;**11**:93-104

[37] Beauchaine TP, Klein DN, Crowell SE, Derbidge C, Gatzke-Kopp L. Multifinality in the development of personality disorders: A biology × sex × environment interaction model of antisocial and borderline traits. Development and Psychopathology. 2009;**21**:735-770

[38] Crowell SE, Beauchaine TP, Linehan MM. A biosocial developmental model of borderline personality: Elaborating and extending Linehan's theory. Psychological Bulletin. 2009;**135**:495-510

[39] Fonagy P, Target M. Attachment Theory and Psychoanalysis. New York: Other Press; 2001

[40] Liotti G. La dimensione interpersonale della coscienza. Roma: Carocci; 1994

[41] Liotti G. Trauma e dissociazione alla luce della teoria dell'attaccamento. Infanzia e adolescenza. 2005;**4**(3):130-144

[42] Liotti G, Fassone G. L'evoluzione delle emozioni e dei sistemi motivazionali. Milano: Raffaello Cortina; 2007

[43] Shore A. Affect Regulation and the Origin of the Self: The Neurobiology of Emotional Development. Mahwah, US: Lawrence Erlbaum Associates; 1994

[44] Shore A. Dysregulation of the right brain: A fundamental mechanism of traumatic attachment and the psychopathogenesis of posttraumatic stress disorder. In: Ardino V, editor. Chapter in Post-Traumatic Stress Disorders in Childhood and Adolescence. Milano: edizioni Unipoli; 2008

[45] Shore A. Bowlby's environment of evolutionary adaptiveness: Recent studies on the interpersonal neurobiology of attachment and emotional development. In: Narvaez D, Panksepp J, Schore A, Gleason T, editors. Evolution, Early Experience, and Human Development: From Research to Practice and Policy. New York: Oxford University Press; 2012. pp. 31-67

[46] Siegel D. The Developing Mind: Toward a Neurobiology of Interpersonal Experience. New York: Guilford Press; 1999

[47] Hill D. Affect Regulation Theory. A Clinical Model. New York: Norton; 2015

[48] Kohut H. How Does Analysis Cure? Chicago: Chicago University Press; 1984

[49] Beebe B, Lachmann F. Infant Research and Adult treatment: Co-Constructing Interactions. Hillsdale, NJ: The Analytic Press; 2002

[50] Beebe B, Lachmann F, Markese S, Buck K, Bahrick L, Chen H, et al. On the origins of disorganized attachment and internal working models: Paper II. An empirical microanalysis of 4-month mother-infant interaction. Psychoanalytic Dialogues. 2012;**22**:352-374

[51] Beck AT, Freeman A, Davis DD. Cognitive Therapy of Personality Disorders. 2nd ed. New York: Guilford Press; 2004

[52] Young JE, Klosko J, Weishaar ME. Schema Therapy: A Practitioner's Guide. New York: Guilford Press; 2003

[53] Linehan MM. Cognitive-Behavioural Treatment of Borderline Personality Disorder. New York: Guilford Press; 1993

[54] Dimaggio G, Semerari A. I disturbi di personalità. Modelli e trattamento: stati mentali, metarappresentazione, cicli interpersonali. Roma: Laterza; 2003

Chapter 5

Recovery, Rehabilitation and Positive Psychology for Chronic Post-Traumatic Stress Disorder: Theoretical and Practical Aspects among French Veterans

Célia Belrose, Lionel Gibert and Marion Trousselard

Abstract

Recovery, in terms of psychological health, is a complex concept that has to be distinguished from the notions of healing and remission. The latter refers to the evolutionary terms of the disease, while recovering from mental illness means to emerge from a psychiatric patient identity and regain an active and satisfying social life. It is clear from the literature that recovery is a complex and elusive concept in a global perspective. Two complementary visions coexist in literature and direct the rehabilitation interventions: a vision focused on mental illness (pathogenic approach) and a vision focused on the concept of sense of subjective well-being and positive mental health (salutogenic approach). Positive psychology studies the conditions, the processes and the actions that contribute to the flourishing or optimal functioning of individuals, groups and institutions. We present results evaluating the psychological resources which remain sustainable for these trauma-exposed soldiers according to their post-traumatic stress disorder (PTSD) symptoms and the dynamics of resource reappropriation after the military rehabilitation program, which focuses on values in action (VIA) as character strengths. They suggest that this approach might bring concepts to better conceptualize the dynamics of recovery and offer levers of action to enrich rehabilitation.

Keywords: recovery, reintegration, positive psychology, post-traumatic stress disorder, veterans

1. Introduction

Recovery is a complex multidimensional concept, which entails at least clinical ("healing", "remission"), mental ("resilience") and socio-behavioural (rehabilitation) dimensions. These dimensions belong to different theoretical fields, and an integration of these complementary approaches about PTSD could be helpful for improving the course of the disorder. At the clinical level, the interchangeable use of the words "healing" and "remission" to mention recovery indicates a confusion of concepts. Whether both "healing" and "remission" target a progressive aspect of the disease, "healing" focuses on the binary outcome of the course of PTSD (sick or cured), whereas "remission" indicates a dynamical process with a risk of coming back in a similar condition at some point in the future.

Recovering from a mental and/or physical disease means, beyond the evolutionary result, to disengage oneself from a patient's identity in order to regain a satisfactory quality of life at the socio-psycho-professional levels. This definition fully enters recovery in the field of positive psychology as this branch of psychology aims at promoting the conditions of an optimal functioning for everyone in a situation of disease or not. The issue of this article is to present the dynamic of recovery and the available conditions for rehabilitation in the light of positive psychology concepts in the specific case of post-traumatic stress disorder (PTSD).

2. The post-traumatic stress disorder

2.1 Definition

PTSD is a debilitating mental disorder that may develop after experiencing or witnessing a life-threatening event. The main characteristics of PTSD are re-experiencing symptoms, avoiding situations that recall the event, increased negative beliefs and feelings and hyperarousal [1]. The recent 11th revision to the World Health Organization's International Classification of Diseases (ICD-11) proposes that PTSD is comprised of three symptom clusters including (i) re-experiencing of the trauma in the here and now, (ii) avoidance of traumatic reminders and (iii) a persistent sense of current threat that is manifested by exaggerated startle and hypervigilance. Furthermore, strong associations are commonly described between PTSD and comorbid conditions, which include depression, substance use disorders and general physical health effects [2, 3]. To be diagnosed with PTSD, a person must experience those symptoms for at least 1 month. Once the symptoms have been observed for 3 months, PTSD is considered as a chronic disorder [1].

PTSD prevalence was found to range from 1 to 7% in Europe [3]. Authors described a prevalence, ranging from 25 to 50% depending on the type of trauma [4]. A prevalence of more than 60% is observed for the direct victims of November 13, 2015 attacks [5]. In the military environment, the prevalence is around 20% according to the violence of the conflicts [6].

The clinical progression, whatever the therapeutic management, shows that (i) more than 20% of the persons are resistant to any treatment [7] and (ii) that around 40% of the persons who recover relapse within the year [8, 9]. With appropriate care, treatment efficiency is variable, and around 20% of the patients do not respond to psychological treatment [7]. On the one hand, there is little research to indicate which treatments are most effective for which patients. For example, whereas significant research to improve treatment for full criteria PTSD exists [7], the evaluation of treatments targeting subclinical PTSD is still in nascent stages [10]. Furthermore, patient treatment preference may affect the differential effectiveness of standardized treatment [11]. On the other hand, a 20-year longitudinal study on a cohort of 214 veterans showed how initial combat stress reaction could lead to volatile chronic stress, with ~40% of recovering subjects relapsing within 1 year of remission [12].

2.2 PTSD: learned mental disability

Unresolved, PTSD can become chronic, causing anguish and suffering in the primary victim and their loved ones. Due to the relatively high prevalence of PTSD in the population, particularly the military, there is an urgent need for treatments that effectively improves recovery. Such statements imply the establishment of an integrated system for the intake of chronic PTSD patients and the evaluation of its impact on the usual impairments of occupational and academic functioning [13–15], marital and family functioning [14, 16], parenting [16, 17] and friendships and socializing [18].

First and foremost, regardless the evolutionary terms of PTSD, it should be highlighted that the traumatic experience deeply transforms the patient. Making everything like it used to be, erasing the trauma, is a rarely feasible wish. Beyond that, the clinical data consider the PTSD as a disease with a high risk of chronic progression. This chronic aspect is expressed by a more or less restrictive but persistent symptomatology or by alternating periods of remission and relapses. Currently, if neither clinical or functional risk factor nor relapse is clearly identified, it is clearly assumed that a stressful environment represents a situational risk factor [6]. So it must be considered that the post-PTSD needs to look at a majority of the patients in a context of a learned mental disability and that this learned disability is expressed by a residual symptomatology and/or by post-traumatic relapse risks.

It has to be noted that the post-traumatic clinical data are numerous and there is no agreed epidemiological data which provide information about the post-traumatic socio-professional experience: how many patients, suffering from a chronic PTSD, do work? Do those who had a job before the onset of the disease frequently lose it? Do they experience great difficulties to keep it when the disease is established? This lack of information is set in recent current events, bearers of a large number of victims of attacks and other acts of terrorism posing the problem of the socio-professional future of these victims as a matter of future public health [10]. It seems necessary to think over the dynamics of the PTSD recovery; to make it feasible, it is important to consider two singular points of the PTSD: (i) the learned mental disability context and (ii) the responsiveness to surroundings, including the one in which the rehabilitation interventions are implemented.

3. The recovery

3.1 Definitions

In 1946, the World Health Organization (WHO) defined in its preamble the notion of health as "a state of complete physical, mental and social well-being and does not merely consist in the absence of illness or infirmity." It therefore requires taking into account the mental and physical health in a comprehensive manner, in order to regain some balance on both a professional and social level.

Thinking over recovery means thinking over the means to allow the sick person to develop and to restore a positive self-image in order to rebuild his/her life despite the limitations imposed by his illness [19, 20]. Recovering from a mental or physical pathology implies becoming autonomous again as far the social professional future is concerned, psychologically getting rid of the identity of being sick in order to regain a mental well-being as a separate individual.

3.2 Approaches for recovery

There are two main approaches of recovery divided into two approaches [21]: (i) a vision focused on the mental disorder (pathogenic) and (ii) a vision focused on the sense of subjective well-being notion or positive mental health (salutogenic).

The pathogenic vision is result-oriented; it deals with assessing the level of recovery for an individual from the result indicators directly and only associated with the disease. This is the most frequent approach among the health professionals, particularly in the field of psychiatry for the chronic progressive mental disorders. This vision is assessed according to a line of action with both poles characterizing the presence versus the absence of the target disease symptoms [19]. It defines rehabilitation interventions targeting healthcare programmes classically defined by the consensual interventions that are designed by the experts to facilitate rehabilitation [20].

The salutogenic vision focuses on the recovery process from the suffering patients' subjective point of view. It characterizes the condition of the sick individual on a positive mental health continuum, which is part of the comprehensive mental health [22]. It is declined according to a well-being/unease axis in terms of emotional, social and psychological resources. The actions referring to it target the set of positive transformations faced by the person along the recovery process and on all the factors that can have a positive or negative impact onto it. These transformations go beyond the frame of the disease and include the optimization of the subjective well-being of the person despite the disease [23].

Taking into account this double dimension of recovery allows to determine a level of clinical severity (pathogenic approach) and of resources (SMP approach) to provide a characterization for the patient's functional ability. This view suggests to think over recovery in terms of functional stages which must be specified according to the targeted mental disorder. For each target, this raises the question of the recovery dynamics based on the assumption that there would be an interdependence of the clinical severity and the resources in the functional by-effects.

3.3 The recovery dynamics

The recovery dynamics is not a linear process. It must be considered as a series of interlinked steps that the patient overcomes at his own pace, with more or less difficulties according to the clinical severity and to the personal and interpersonal resources. The relations maintained by the patient with his emotional and medical support are essential for this dynamics, and the previous negative medical experiences are widely acknowledged as obstacles in the recovery process [24].

It has been proposed that recovery process should implicate six steps [23] (**Table 1**):

i. A so-called standstill step characterized by a feeling of deep despair resulting in a withdrawal position of the individual.

ii. An awareness step that corresponds to the emergence of a sense of fight against fatality. It reflects the recovered control of a personal feeling of action and the emergence of a possible projection in the future.

iii. A preparation step along which the individual reviews his/her forces and his/her weaknesses to achieve it.

iv. A rebuilding step which means an active work to define targets and to revive the altered self-determination in order to restore a positive self-image. It deals with maintaining an active acceptance of the disease allowing the patient to reconnect with his/her personal identity.

v. A preparation step throughout which the patient evaluates the personal and interpersonal lever implementation modalities he/she has to allow the "development" step.

vi. The last "development" step demonstrates the culmination of resilience mechanisms. "The resilience represents the set of protective factors, of processes and mechanisms which contribute to a successful outcome despite the exposure to stressors known to cause a significant risk to the development of a mental disorder" [25].

This last stage characterizes the condition of a patient able to live independently a satisfactory life.

Thinking over the recovery dynamics, regardless the proposed models and stages, suggests to think over the patients' capacities of resilience, not in terms of a patient's trajectory prediction but of personal journey. This journey is the experience of the patient's recovery, per se. The rhetoric of the patient proposes an accessible entry point to this subjective experience. A better characterization of personal, family and social protective factors which support the journey will contribute to define which modalities are the more able to sustain a favourable outcome when exposed to adversity.

3.4 Recovery and PTSD

Faced to the psychological changes when PTSD, there are several questions to understand for improving recovery.

A first question deals with the resources which remain sustainable for these patients. A systematic appraisal of the positive mental health during the clinical diagnose would be a first step. Is there any resources reappropriation dynamics likely to be characterized? In other words, do some resources represent better levers likely to be support candidates to initiate the way to recovery? Is it also necessary to evaluate whether the still available positive resources are linked to the clinical severity despite the psychological trauma? These questions are to be considered both for the patients responding to treatment and for those who progress towards a chronic PTSD.

Answering these questions is an absolute prerequisite to build rehabilitation pathways adapted to the available patients' resources profiles with a focus on the resources, which could be optimized. It is necessary to develop prospective studies to define some operational psychological markers along the path towards recovery. The markers should take into account not only the learned disability situational determinants, to identify the existential issues of "living with a disability", but also the resources to overcome it. Having such tools will then allow to define actions suitable to patients and to assess their added value in the PTSD patient's recovery.

Steps	Description
1. Standstill step	The patient feels of deep despair
2. Awareness step	The patient recovers the feeling of a control in his/her action with a possible projection in the future
3. Preparation step	The patient reviews his/her forces and his/her weaknesses to achieve it
4. Rebuilding step	The patient actively works to define targets and to revive the altered self-determination in order to restore a positive self-image
5. Preparation step	The patient evaluates the personal and interpersonal lever implementation modalities he/she has to allow the "development" step
6. Development step	The patient is implied in resilience dynamic

Table 1.
Six steps of the recovery [23].

4. Mental health rehabilitation

4.1 Definitions

The rehabilitation is defined as "a set of therapeutic interventions enabling the person's potential while giving him/her back the power to improve his/her life" [26]. The mission of psychiatric rehabilitation is to assist persons with long-term psychiatric disabilities increase their functioning, so they are successful and satisfied in the environments of their choice with the least amount of ongoing professional intervention. It is at the heart of the recovery process and applies the principles and objectives of this process in a concrete way. Six main objectives can be identified: (i) reduce the symptoms, (ii) reinforce the family support and the network, (iii) reduce discrimination and stigmatization, (iv) improve the social skills, (v) reduce the negative results of an intervention or a hospitalization and (vi) encourage the power to act while improving the self-determination and the self-perception. Reaching these objectives, in fine, leads to develop interventions supporting the patient throughout a conscious journey towards a purpose that is not based upon his/her healing but upon his/her well-being and his/her functionality.

It deals with how to recover a full rich life for oneself after a functional alteration by redefining a new function for oneself. From a practical standpoint, psychiatric rehabilitation can be done through clinical interventions, specifically aiming at developing abilities and support interventions. The SAMSHA's National Registry of Evidence-Based Programs and Practices recommends that the different actors involved have a practical and theoretical knowledge base, facilitating attitudes and values as well as abilities fostering a strong therapeutic alliance [27]. For the services implementing it, they pose the need for a collaborative, patient-focused and individualized functioning [26, 28]. It relies on probative experimental data to define the best clinical practice and the psychopathological scope. These elements make of psychiatric rehabilitation a field of research and practice [29].

4.2 Positive psychology and rehabilitation

Psychiatric rehabilitation is developing while integrating in its interventions some tools aiming at "spreading and developing" positive resources which are part of positive psychology field of studies [30, 31]. In particular, the interventions are based on "mindfulness" [32] and on reorienting the intention towards the positive aspects of life (inspired by the researches in the field of positive psychology) [33]. They have thus developed in order to improve the individuals' well-being, their flourishing level and their adaption capacity. These interventions are witnessing a growing interest in the scientific literature [33, 34] in the light of their positive impact on well-being. These benefits concern the subjective well-being, defined by a high frequency of positive effects, a low frequency of negative aspects and a high level of satisfaction in terms of quality of one's life [35, 36], but also the psychological well-being which includes the self-acceptance, the sense of autonomy, the quality of relationships, the level of flourishing and the sense of one's environment control, as well as considering that life makes sense [37]. If the interventions that include positive psychology approaches primarily target the salutogenic axis of recovery, they also induce the development and/or the regain of a cognitive functioning, which is part of the resilience process.

They promote a spread attention, leading to a flexible and creative thought, and they boost social, physical and psychological to deal with the different issues related to disease [30]. Currently, these interventions have been successful in the optimization of performance (cognitive and sports performance) and in the management of professional stressors (psychosocial risks). They begin in the field of rehabilitation. Studies targeting the role played by the optimal experience (state of intense concentration, of commitment, of situation control and of clarity of the objectives, associated to a positive emotional state) in the personal growth have been carried out in the field of mental health [38]. A longitudinal study conducted on a patient who had developed an anxiety disorder has notably shown that a therapy aiming at identifying and cultivating optimal activities contributes to reduce symptomatology [39]. It has also been observed that in the case of physical pains with a disability that occurred during teenage years or as an adult, a very specific phenomenon called *optimal experience transformation* [40]: the disability that arose does not prevent the individual from continuing to cultivate the optimal activities he used to practice before, unless some limits, due to his new physical condition, force him to stop or to give up these activities forever. In the latter case, to keep on living optimal experiences, the person can decide to modify the activities he/she used to practice before by adapting them to his new physical condition; he/she can replace them or ad new activities and look for new fields in which he/she could engage and develop his/her abilities. Thus, developing optimal experience supports the promotion of the well-being with at least two lines of action: contributing to help the person to recover his/her physical and social functioning during the process of rehabilitation and/or contributing to the building of a new commitment in life focused on the emergence of new interests [41, 42]. These studies also reflect the interest in setting up interventions in positive psychology for the rehabilitation actors; not only does it deal with fostering their health protection but also with fostering the conditions of a therapeutic alliance efficiently supporting the steps for rehabilitation [42]. Lastly, positive psychology has developed and validated numerous psychometric tools in the field of positive health [43]. A correctly proper use in a protocol of rehabilitation appears to be necessary to get a rigorous evaluation of the interventions and of their dynamics. This use must take into account not only the individuals (patients and rehabilitation actors) but also their interaction in terms of therapeutic alliance.

4.3 Psychiatric rehabilitation and PTSD

The western armies have developed programmes of psychiatric rehabilitation for the veterans with systematized assessments. Regardless of the interventions carried out, the transfer to the civil environment is difficult, especially because the duration of the developed programmes is limited in the sense that they fit into a time window determined by the military institution of the country and the military's status. In the case of civilians suffering from PTSD, there are few studies about recovery, and there is no community of practice of psychiatric rehabilitation.

In positive psychology, the concept of post-traumatic growth (PTG) has been proposed [44–46]. This field of research takes an interest in the links between serious life events (often sources of major crisis for the individuals suffering or not from PTSD) and the positive psychological changes. Not only has the person survived a situation putting at stake the question of his/her own survival (accident, natural disaster, serious disease, etc.), he/she has also experienced major and positive inner changes in fields as varied as the appreciation of others, of one's intimacy and/or of life. This concept directly targets the experience of individuals whose development has surpassed what they were before the crisis. Some researchers suggest that the PTG following adversity represents a natural normal and natural process and that each of us has been provided with an inner and innate dynamics (capacity for endurance); to reach it, it sometimes has to be stimulated, guided or accompanied [45, 46].

So, the potentiation of growth as a goal for the therapeutic activity is of growing interest. However, within the context of the PTSD, the relationship between the severity of PTSD and the PTG seems to follow a curvilinear rather than linear curve [44]. When the level of post-traumatic stress increases, the level of post-traumatic development also rises. But beyond a certain threshold, the level of development seems to drop.

5. Towards a positive psychiatric rehabilitation

Positive psychology groups the set of studies together under one heading concerning comprehension and optimization of the human potential [31]. It targets the individual and interpersonal levers but also groups and institutional levers to study the dynamics of positive changes at the individual and collective level. At the individual level, it aims at better understanding the building mechanisms of the subjective experiences (e.g., well-being—in the past), of the optimal experiences (for the present) and of optimism (for the future). It is de facto intended for any individual in his life environment, whether he/she is suffering or not from physical and/or psychic disease. This approach supports an autonomous conception of recovery in the psychic disability, free of the medical model. It targets three main determinants of the recovery potential:

i. The perception of autonomy defined as a cognitive source resulting from the interaction between inner positive resources (dispositions for being mindful, motivation and optimism contributing to personality) and "coping" resources (contributing to adaptation strategies).

ii. The experiential dimension (subjective experience of the disability) but also the respect of his autonomy of action. These determinants require taking into account the "first person" patient's point of view.

iii. The reversibility of the dependence relationships between illness, disabilities and social disadvantage has to be taken into account.

This characteristic of the psychic disability has practical implications: when bringing an improvement in the consequences of the illness, in the social disadvantage that it induces (e.g., social isolation), it is permissible to expect in return a benefit on certain disabilities to support the recovery and in fine on the illness itself [30].

The recovery process implicates four axes for changes [47]: (i) finding and keeping hope (believing in oneself, personal feeling of being able to take action, being optimistic), (ii) finding a positive restored identity (having a new identity with the illness while keeping a positive self-image), (iii) giving meaning to one's new life and (iv) controlling one's life (taking back control of one's life). These changes appear to be echoed with the notion of health behaviours reinforced by practicing mindfulness exercises. Three salutogenic health behaviours are developed/reinforced by the practice of mindfulness [48]: intention, attention and attitude. Intention is associated with the medical care compliance as it is observed through the constancy in mindfulness practice and along the training: the persons who engaged themselves in mindfulness tend to be more conscientious [49, 50] and to keep going in this direction [50, 51]. Attention aims at developing skills to remain focused on an object (body, breathing) in the present moment [52]. It fosters a non-elaborative consciousness about thoughts, emotions and perceived sensations. This allows not to be captured by negative effects and to cultivate one's resources [53]. The attitude developed by the mindfulness practice finally insists on a trend towards experience leading to a cognitive curiosity allowing to open one's mind to new experiences [51]. It is set up in a non-judgmental attitude enabling an acceptation with a clear conscience. It is a lever for taking into account health advice and environmental supports. These three main behaviours developed thanks to mindfulness result in a change of perspective enabling to recapture positive resources. Taking into account the mechanism of an individual's positive changes which positive psychology focuses on understanding constitutes a prerequisite for the development of rehabilitation programmes targeting the valorization, the reinforcement and/or the recapturing of individual potential. This view allows to reinforce the health behaviours which are essential to maintaining the recovery dynamics. It integrates each individual's uniqueness to support the recovery process towards discovering a new meaning and a new goal for one's life.

6. Some results

In light of the psychological changes in an individual suffering from chronic post-traumatic stress disorder, questions are being raised in order to understand and facilitate recovery and a return to work. This is particularly challenging for soldiers suffering from chronic PTSD. A French military rehabilitation program proposes the broadening of the relationships between recovery and reintegration by incorporating approaches from the field of positive psychology for soldiers with chronic PTSD. The aim of the study was to evaluate (i) the psychological resources which remain sustainable for these trauma-exposed soldiers according to their PTSD symptoms; (ii) the dynamics of resource reappropriation after the military rehabilitation program, which focuses on values in action as character strengths; and (iii) how these resources and their reappropriation facilitate civilian professional reintegration.

We conducted a prospective study with 56 trauma-exposed soldiers with a clinical diagnosis of chronic PTSD [54]. PTSD severity and psychological resources (optimism, mindfulness, well-being, motivation, self-esteem and VIA) were assessed before and after the rehabilitation program. After the identification of resource profiles, we analysed the impact of the program on resource levels and successful reintegration into a civilian job.

Three profiles were identified based on the psychological resources of the soldiers. Profiles 1, 2 and 3 differed in terms of clinical severity (PCL5). Profile 1 exhibited both the highest level of resources and the lowest clinical severity of PTSD but did not modify its resources after the intervention program when compared to profile 3. Profile 3 was characterized by the lowest level of resources, the highest clinical severity of PTSD and the highest reappropriation in all VIAs. This profile was associated with the highest rate of reintegration success 1 year after the intervention.

7. Conclusions

The temporality of the rebuilding is set in a complex progression in which technology differs depending on the individuals. It is a "fundamentally personal and unique process aiming at changing one's attitudes, one's values, one's feelings, one's goals, one's skills and one's missions. It is a way of living a satisfying life full of hope and a productive life despite the limits resulting from the illness (...)" [53].

If the recovery experience is personal to the individual, positive psychology targets generic resources and develops interventions to reinforce them. Its development in the context of the chronic illness should contribute to better define the actions to implement and their temporality.

Acknowledgements

The authors wish to thank the "Cellule d'Aide aux Blessés de l'Armée de Terre" and the associations of the "Gueules Cassées" and "Terre—Fraternité" for their financial support.

Author details

Célia Belrose[1,2,3], Lionel Gibert[1,3,4] and Marion Trousselard[1,2,3,5]*

1 Département de neurosciences et Sciences Cognitives, Brétigny sur Orge Cedex, France

2 APEMAC-EPSam UDL UFR SHS, Metz Cedex 1, France

3 Réseau abc des psychotraumas, France

4 Centre Hospitalier Paul Guiraud, Villejuif, France

5 Ecole du Val de Grâce, Paris, France

*Address all correspondence to: marion.trousselard@gmail.com

References

[1] American Psychiatric Association. Diagnostic and Statistical Manual of Mental Disorder. 5th ed. Washington, DC: Elsevier; 2013

[2] Hoge CW, Terhakopian A, Castro CA, Messer SC, Engel CC. Association of posttraumatic stress disorder with somatic symptoms, health care visits, and absenteeism among Iraq war veterans. American Journal of Psychiatry. 2007;**164**(1):150-153. DOI: 10.1176/ajp.2007.164.1.150

[3] Kessler RC, Chiu WT, Demler O, Merikangas KR, Walters EE. Prevalence, severity, and comorbidity of 12-month DSM-IV disorders in the National Comorbidity Survey Replication. Archives of General Psychiatry. 2005;**62**(6):617-627. DOI: 10.1001/archpsyc.62.6.617

[4] Yehuda R, Hoge CW, McFarlane AC, Vermetten E, Lanius RA, Nievergelt CM, et al. Hyman SE. Post-traumatic stress disorder. Nature Reviews. Disease Primers 2015;**1**:15057. DOI: 10.1038/nrdp.2015.57

[5] Gibert L, El Hage W, Tarquinio C, Fallissard B, Trousselard M. Paris terrorist attacks: Post-traumatic stress disorder risk factors inform care guidance. European Journal of Trauma and Dissociation. 2015. (in press). Available online: September 5, 2018. Available from: https://doi.org/doi:10.1016/j.ejtd.2018.08.003

[6] Zvolensky MJ, Kotov R, Schechter CB, Gonzalez A, Vujanovic A, Pietrzak RH, et al. Post-disaster stressful life events and WTC-related posttraumatic stress, depressive symptoms, and overall functioning among responders to the World Trade Center. Journal of Psychiatric Research. 2015;**61**:97-105. DOI: 10.1016/j.jpsychires.2014.11.010

[7] Zohar J, Juven-Wetzler A, Sonnino R, Cwikel-Hamzany S, Balaban E, Cohen H. New insights into secondary prevention in post-traumatic stress disorder. Dialogues in Clinical Neuroscience. 2011;**13**:301-309

[8] Spaniol L, Bellingham R, Cohen B, Spaniol S. The Recovery Workbook. II: Connectedness. Center for Psychiatric Rehabilitation, Sargent College of Health and Rehabilitation Sciences. Boston MA, United States: Boston University; 2003

[9] Tarrier N, Sommerfield C, Pilgrim H, Humphreys L. Cognitive therapy or imaginal exposure in the treatment of post-traumatic stress disorder. Twelve-month follow-up. The British Journal of Psychiatry. 1999;**175**:571-575. DOI: 10.1192/bjp.175.6.571

[10] Korte KJ, Allan NP, Gros DF, Acierno R. Differential treatment response trajectories in individuals with subclinical and clinical PTSD. Journal of Anxiety Disorder. 2016;**38**:95-101. DOI: 10.1016/j.janxdis.2016.01.006

[11] Zoellner LA, Roy-Byrne PP, Mavissakalian M, Feeny NC. Doubly randomized preference trial of prolonged exposure versus sertraline for treatment of PTSD. American Journal of Psychiatry. 2019;**176**(4):287-296. DOI: 10.1176/appi.ajp.2018.17090995

[12] Salomon Z, Mikulincer M. Trajectories of PTSD: A 20-year longitudinal study. American Journal of Psychiatry. 2006;**163**(4):659-666. DOI: 10.1176/appi.ajp.163.4.659

[13] Bolton D, Hill J, O'Ryan D, Udwin O, Boyle S, Yule W. Long-term effects of psychological trauma on psychosocial functioning. Journal of Child Psychology and Psychiatry. 2004;**45**(5):1007-1014

[14] Rona RJ, Jones M, Iversen A, Hull L, Greenberg N, Fear NT, et al. The impact of posttraumatic stress

disorder on impairment in the UK military at the time of the Iraq war. Journal of Psychiatry Research. 2009;**43**(6):649-655. DOI: 10.1016/j.jpsychires.2008.09.006

[15] Smith MW, Schnurr PP, Rosenheck RA. Employment outcomes and PTSD symptom severity. Mental Health Services Research. 2005;7(2):89-101. DOI: 10.1007/s11020-005-3780-2

[16] Cohen E, Zerach G, Solomon Z. The implication of combat-induced stress reaction, PTSD, and attachment in parenting among war veterans. Journal of Family Psychology. 2011;**25**(5):688-698. DOI: 10.1037/a0024065

[17] Solomon Z, Debby-Aharon S, Zerach G, Horesh D. Marital adjustment, parental functioning, and emotional sharing in war veterans. Journal of Family Issues. 2011;**32**(1):127-147. DOI: 10.1177/0192513X10379203

[18] Laffaye C, Cavella S, Drescher K, Rosen C. Relationships among PTSD symptoms, social support, and support source in veterans with chronic PTSD. Journal of Traumatic Stress. 2008;**21**(4):394-401. DOI: 10.1002/jts.20348

[19] Davidson L, Roe D. Recovery from versus recovery in serious mental illness: One strategy for lessening confusion plaguing recovery. Journal of Mental Health. 2007;**16**(4):459-470. DOI: 10.1080/09638230701482394

[20] Unité d'évaluation des technologies et des modes d'intervention en santé [Health Technology Assessment and Intervention Unit]. Les meilleures pratiques cliniques en réadaptation psychosociale (ET31-0606). [Best Clinical Practice in Psychosocial Rehabilitation]. Institut universitaire en santé mentale de Québec; 2015

[21] Provencher HL, Keyes CLM. Complete mental health recovery: Bridging mental illness with positive mental health. Journal of Public Mental Health. 2011;**10**(1):54-66. DOI: 10.1108/17465721111134556

[22] Benny M, Lalonde JA, Landry-Cuerrier L, Marinier L, Sergerie MA, Huot A. Santé mentale et psychopathologie, une approche biopsychosociale (2nd ed.). [Mental Health and Psychopathology, a Biopsychosocial Approach]. Québec: Modulo; 2016

[23] Andresen R, Caputi P, Oades L. Stages of recovery instrument: Development of a measure of recovery from serious mental illness. Australian and New Zealand Journal of Psychiatry. 2006;**40**:972-980. DOI: 10.1080/j.1440-1614.2006.01921.x

[24] Hjemdal O, Friborg O, Stiles TC, Rosenvinge JH, Martinussen M. Resilience predicting psychiatric symptoms: A prospective study in adjustment to stressful life events. Clinical Psychology & Psychotherapy. 2006;**13**:194-201. DOI: 10.1002/cpp.488

[25] Legay D. Les pratiques françaises de réadaptation sociale : Les patients schizophrènes. [The French practices of psychosocial rehabilitation: Therapeutic systems for schizophrenic patients]. L'Information Psychiatrique. 2002;77:259-263

[26] Farkas M, Anthony W. Psychiatric rehabilitation interventions: A review. International Review of Psychiatry. 2010;**22**(2):114-129. DOI: 10.3109/09540261003730372

[27] SAMSHA's National Registry of Evidence based Programs and Practices. U.S. Department of Health and Human Services, Substance Abuse and Mental Health Services Administration [Internet]. 2014. Available from: www.nrepp.samhsa.gov/ViewIntervention.aspx?id=241 [Accessed: March 02, 2019]

[28] Tempier R, Favrod J. Réadaptation psychiatrique en milieu francophone: Pratiques actuelles, défis futurs. [psychiatric rehabilitation in a French-speaking setting: Current practices, future challenges]. Canadian Journal of Psychiatry. 2002;**47**(7):621-627. DOI: 10.1177/070674370204700703

[29] Reed GM, Leornardi M, Ayuso-Mateos JL, Materzanini A, Castronuovo D, Manara A, et al. Implementing the ICF in psychiatry rehabilitation setting for people with serious mental illness in the Lombardy region of Italy. Disability and Rehabilitation. 2009;**31**(S1):S170-S173. DOI: 10.3109/09638280903317955

[30] Fredrickson BL. The broaden- and -build theory of positive emotions. Philosophical Transactions of the Royal Society of London. Series B, Biological Sciences. 2004;**359**:1367-1377. DOI: 10.1098/rstb.2004.1512

[31] Seligman MEP, Csikszentmihalyi M. Positive psychology: An introduction. American Journal of Psychology. 2000;**35**:5-14. DOI: 10.1037/0003-066X.55.1.5

[32] Chiesa A, Serretti A. Mindfulness-based stress reduction for stress management in healthy people: A review and meta-analysis. Journal of Alternative and Complementary Medicine. 2009;**15**(5):593-600. DOI: 10.1089/acm.2009.0546

[33] Sin NL, Lyubomirsky S. Enhancing well-being and alleviating depressive symptoms with positive psychology interventions: A practice-friendly meta-analysis. Journal of Clinical Psychology. 2009;**65**(5):467-487. DOI: 10.1002/jclp.20593

[34] Kashdan T, Ciarrochi J. Mindfulness, Acceptance, and Positive Psychology: The Seven Foundations of Well-Being. Oakland, United States: Context Press, New Harbinger Publications; 2013

[35] Diener E. Subjective well-being. Psychological Bulletin. 1994;**95**:542-575

[36] Ryff CD. Happiness is everything, or is it: Explorations on the meaning of psychological well-being. Journal of Personality and Social Psychology. 1989;**57**:1069-1081

[37] Delle Fave AA. Life worth living. Contributions to positive psychology. In: Csikszentmihalyi M, Csikszentmihalyi I, editors. The Impact of Subjective Experience on the Quality of Life. A Central Issue for Health Professionals. New York: Oxford University Press; 2006. pp. 165-181

[38] Delle Fave A, Massinimi F. Experience sampling method and the measuring of clinical change: A case of axiety syndrome. In: deVries MW, editor. The Experience of Psychopathology. Cambridge: Cambridge University Press; 1992. pp. 280-298

[39] Bassi M, Delle Fave A. Dimensions of well-being. Research and intervention. In: DelleFave A, editor. The Daily Experience of Italian Adolescents' in Family Interactions. Gender and Developmental Issues. Milan: Franco Angeli; 2006. pp. 172-190

[40] Delle Fave A, Massimini F. Bringing subjectivity into focus: Optimal experiences, life themes, and person-centered rehabilitation. In: Linley PA, Joseph S, editors. Positive Psychology in Practice. New York: Wiley; 2004. pp. 581-597

[41] Joseph S, Linley A. Positive Therapy: A Meta-Theory for Positive Psychological Practice. New York: Routledge; 2006

[42] Kretsch M, Tarquinio C, Joseph S, Martin-Krumm C. Traité de psychologie positive. In: Martin-Krumm C, Tarquinio C, editors. Psychologie Positive et Développement/Croissance

Post-Traumatique : Changements Positifs et Bénéfices Perçus Suite Aux Evènements de Vie Graves [Positive Psychology and Post Traumatic Development/Growth: Positive Changes and Perceived Benefits of Serious Life Events]. Bruxelles: DeBoeck; 2011. pp. 401-423

[43] Shankland R, Martin-Krumm C. Les outils d'évaluation en Psychologie Positive. [Assessment tools in positive psychology]. Pratiques Psychologiques. 2012;**18**:171-187. DOI: 10.1016/j.prps.2012.02.004

[44] Butler LD, Blasey CM, Garlan RW, McCaslin SE, Azarow J, Chen XH, et al. Posttraumatic growth following the terrorist attacks of September 11, 2001: Cognitive, coping, and trauma symptom predictors in an internet convenience sample. Traumatology. 2005;**11**(4):247-267. DOI: 10.1177/153476560501100405

[45] Calhoun LG, Tedeschi RG. Meaning reconstruction and the experience of loss. In: Neymeyer RA, editor. Posttraumatic Growth: Positive Lessons of Loss. Washington, DC: American Psychological Association; 2001. pp. 157-172

[46] Tedeschi RG, Calhoun LG. Trauma and Transformation: Growing in the Aftermath of Suffuring. Thousand Oaks, CA: Sage; 1995. p. 175. DOI: 10.4135/9781483326931

[47] Andresen R, Oades L, Caputi P. The experience from recovery schizophrenia: Towards an empirically validated stage model. Australian and New Zeeland Journal of Psychiatry. 2003;**37**:586-594. DOI: 10.1046/j.1440-1614.2003.01234.x

[48] Shapiro S, Carlson LE, Astin JA, Freedman B. Mechanism of mindfulness. Journal of Clinical Psychology. 2006;**62**(3):373-386. DOI: 10.1002/jclp.20237

[49] Bishop SR, Lau M, Shapiro S, Carlson L, Anderson ND, Carmody J, et al. Mindfulness: A proposed operational definition. Clinical Psychology: Science and Practice. 2004;**11**:230-241. DOI: 10.1093/clipsy.bph077

[50] van den Hurk P, Wings T, Giommi F, Barendregt HP, Speckens A, van Schie H. On the relationship between the practice of mindfulness meditation and personality: An exploratory analysis of the mediating role of mindfulness skills. Mindfulness. 2011;**2**:194-200. DOI: 10.1007/s12671-011-0060-7

[51] Nyklíček I, Kuijpers KF. Effects of mindfulness-based stress reduction intervention on psychological well-being quality of life: Is increased mindfulness indeed the mechanism? Annals of Behavioral Medicine. 2008;**35**:331-340. DOI: 10.1007/s12160-008-9030-2

[52] Rosenzweig S, Greeson JM, Reibel DK, Green JS, Jasser SA, Beasley D. Mindfulness-based stress reduction for chronic pain conditions: Variation in treatment outcomes role of home meditation practice. Journal of Psychosomatic Research. 2010;**68**:29-36. DOI: 10.1016/j.jpsychores.2009.03.010

[53] Anthony WA. Recovery from mental illness: The guiding vision of the mental health service system in the 1990's. Psychosocial Rehabilitation Journal. 1993;**16**(4):11-23

[54] Belrose C, Duffaud A, Dutheil F, Trichereau J, Trousselard M. Challenges associated with the civilian reintegration of soldiers with chronic PTSD: A new approach integrating psychological resources and values in action reappropriation. Frontiers in Psychiatry. 2019;**9**:737. DOI: 10.3389/fpsyt.2018.00737

Section 3

Psychological Trauma - Different Treatment Aspects

Chapter 6

The Role of Therapeutic Landscape in Improving Mental Health of People with PTSD

Shima Taheri, Amirhosein Shabani and Maryam Ghasemi Sichani

Abstract

Post-traumatic stress disorder (PTSD) as a complex disorder, with serious consequences, affects the quality of life of the individual, the family, as well as the community. Therefore, the subject of this chapter is to study how to reduce stress and improve the quality of life of these people and consequently the community. This chapter is based on documentary studies including the foundations of the theory, the study of the results of experiments in the world, and case studies in this field, which shows that the interaction of individuals with PTSD and therapeutic landscapes can act as a therapeutic mechanism. In the following, features from therapeutic landscapes that help to optimize mental health levels are reviewed in people with PTSD, briefly.

Keywords: mental health, therapeutic landscape, PTSD, stress, physical space, nature

1. Introduction

Stress control improves health, prevents diseases, enhances the quality of life, and reduces health costs [1]. To date, little research has been conducted on the positive and negative effects of the physical environment for people with post-traumatic stress disorder (PTSD), and in particular, little is known about what types of outdoor spaces, and what elements and activities in those outdoor spaces, will be of greatest benefit. The complex combination of physical and neurological injuries interwoven with long-lasting emotional challenges may call for unique design concepts [2]. The notable point about research on quality of life and improving the health of people with PTSD is that so far, many studies have been done about them, however, few studies have been conducted on the role of therapeutic landscape in improving the health of people with PTSD, since this object is a very important disorder that can affect the overall life of a person and affect the work, psychosocial, and physical activity, so that stress relief is highly effective in determining the effectiveness of healthcare and rehabilitation. This chapter first gives a brief overview of PTSD and its levels and attributes then investigates the foundations of the theory and philosophy of association with the nature and effects of nature on health in therapeutic landscape form; the next section is about therapeutic landscapes backgrounds for people with PTSD; also, we discuss the need for a therapeutic landscape to improve the health of people with PTSD and finally introduce some effective environmental factors in the effectiveness of the therapeutic landscape for PTSD.

2. PTSD

Trauma exposure leads to various psychiatric disorders including depression, anxiety, bipolar disorders, personality disorders, psychotic disorders, and trauma-related disorders, especially post-traumatic stress disorder [3]. Post-traumatic stress disorder is classified in the new class of traumatic and stress disorder [4]. The term post-traumatic stress disorder was first coined in the 1970s to replace post-Vietnam syndrome. The condition was formally recognized in 1980 in the DSM-IV [5].

PTSD generally appears within 3 months after a traumatic experience such as sexual or psychological abuse or assault, a serious accident, natural disaster, or war-related event(s) [6] or a non-war traumatic event such as a terrorist attack, family violence, and serious injury [7]. It often occurs with—and may be exacerbated by or contribute to—related disorders, including depression [8, 9] substance abuse [10], memory loss, and other physical, mental health problems, and suicidal ideation [11, 12]. Although the majority of PTSD cases in the US are caused by non-combat trauma [13, 14], the lifetime prevalence of the disorder is higher in combat-exposed cases [15].

Individuals with PTSD continue to experience the psychological effects of trauma, including re-experiencing symptoms, avoidance of similar stimuli, negative cognition and mood, and increased physical arousal, long after being removed to a safe environment [7]. They may also suffer a wide range of consequences of revealing their problems, such as a higher likelihood of losing jobs or being discriminated against in the workplace, social exclusion, lower income, difficulties in renting residences, exclusion from social communities, and legal difficulties [16]. In addition to the patients themselves, family members, friends, community members, colleagues, and employers are also indirectly affected by PTSD. Currently, more than 2% of the US population (about 7.7 million people) is known to suffer from PTSD, and 8–9% of the US population reports experiencing lifetime PTSD [17].

More than 60% of men and 51% of women face a major stressful event during their lifetime [18, 19]. Of course, the prevalence of PTSD in the typical population is reported to be between 5 and 10% [20, 21], which shows that only a small group of people with a major incident eventually have PTSD [22] which, of course, is highly dependent on stress. According to the World Health Organization, 450 million people in the world are suffering from vascular and psychiatric illness [23]. About 65% of patients with mental disorders live with their families [24]. The overall prevalence of PTSD is about 8% in general, which is 10–12% in women and 5–6% in men. Also, the prevalence of diseases associated with PTSD is high, with about two-thirds of these patients having at least two other disorders [25, 26]. Over 40% of the risk for PTSD may be genetically heritable [27]. Post-traumatic stress disorder (PTSD) stands out as a major mental illness and is becoming a serious public health challenge.

3. The role of nature in improving physical and mental health

In health geography and environmental psychology, substantial literatures on green space environments emphasize their potential to promote health and well-being [28–31]. Fortunately, there is a recently rediscovered body of evidence that supports the view that nature generally, and everyday living environments in particular, can have a profound effect on health and well-being. Connecting with nature can restore cognitive attention [32, 33], improve blood pressure and self-esteem [34], support pro-environmental behaviors [35], decrease symptoms of attention deficit disorder [36], and improve community resilience [37]. Contact with nature is an effective "upstream health promotion" tool for whole populations. That is, it is useful in prevention of mental health conditions [38]. Studies have shown that exposure to natural environments enhances our ability to recover from stress, illness, and injury, and provides a wide range of social, psychological, and physiological benefits [39, 40]. Across our towns and cities, a connection with nature has been found to be a vital, albeit often unconscious, part of being human.

In the late 1970s, the environmental psychologist Ulrich began research on the emotional and psychological effects of environmental esthetics on individuals with a special experience in terms of psychological challenges. In 1984, his paper, "The View through a window" can be effective in restoring the patient after surgery," posed a serious discussion about access to nature in hospitals, which was published in the journal Science. The outcomes data revealed that patients with the nature view had shorter hospital stays, suffered fewer postsurgical complications, needed fewer doses of potent narcotic pain medication, and received more positive written comments in their medical records from staff [41].

Ulrich's study, cited in thousands of publications—from books to scholarly journals to newspaper and magazine articles—was, and continues to be, signify for two reasons. First, it demonstrated to the medical community—using the same empirical, quantitative methods that they used and respected—that the physical environment, and specifically views of nature, had a measurable positive effect on patient health. Second, it established a business case for providing access to nature. All of the improved health outcomes for patients—duration of hospital stay, amount of pain medication, degree of strain on nursing staff, and level of patient satisfaction—translated directly to potential cost savings [6].

Physical settings can play a role in coping with stress; in particular, experimental research has found strong evidence between exposure to natural environments and recovery from physiological stress and mental fatigue, giving support to both "stress recovery theory" and "attention restoration theory" [42–44]. In fact, exposure to natural environments protects people against the impact of environmental stressors and offer physiological, emotional, and attention restoration more so than urban environments. Natural places that allow the renewal of personal adaptive resources to meet the demands of everyday life are called "restorative environments." Natural environments elicit greater calming responses than urban environments, and in relation to their vision there is a general reduction of physiological symptoms of stress. Exposure to natural scenes mediates the negative effects of stress reducing the negative mood state and above all enhancing positive emotions. Moreover, one can recover the decrease of cognitive performance associated with stress, especially reflected in attention tasks, through the salutary effect of viewing nature. Giving the many benefits of contact with nature, plans for urban environments should attend to restrictiveness [45].

The neuroscientist Esther Sternberg suggests that part of nature's benefit is derived from the multitude of simultaneous positive sensory experiences [46, 47]. Proximity to nature, especially trees, was also found to have a beneficial effect on the amount of domestic violence in Chicago public housing households [48], women's ability to cope with major life issues [49], and amount of inner-city crime [50].
A study by team of Li [51] showed that nature therapy increases the activity of natural lethal cells that are part of the immune system against cancer risk. This in turn

helps to increase resistance to stress. Past research demonstrates that naturalistic settings may offer benefits in terms of stress reduction and improved mental states within corrections environments [52].

4. Theoretical and philosophical foundation

In stress reduction theory, Ulrich is emphasized on health positive results by reducing stress based on two main reasons. First, many people who are ill or caring for a patient experience stress. Second, many people-someone who are not aware of this sign-are demanding environments in order to reduce stress where is predominant in nature [53]. There is powerful evidence that indicates (1) sensory control, (2) social support, (3) physical movement, (4) natural positive distractions help reduce stress [44, 54, 55].

Attention restoration theory was developed by Rachel and Stephen Kaplan in the decade 1980 in their book "Nature Experience: One Psychological Approach" was introduced to describe environmental impacts [32, 56] on humans and emphasizes the role of the natural environment for the physical, psychological recovery of the individual as a factor in the restoration of thought. According to this view, placing in the environment can reduce people's psychological pressure and improve the fatigue of the audience. This theory claims that people after spending time in nature, or even looking at the scenes of nature can focus better. The natural range is with many soft charms that a person can show in "simple and instant attention," such as moving clouds across the sky, the sound of leaves in mild wind, or the sound of flowing water in a stream full of rock. Kaplan's theory defines two-related systems: directed attention, engaging in a particular task, which is often difficult and stressful (like taking a test, doing surgery), requires simultaneous removal of the sensory stimulus. Psychological restoration can be described as the ability to perceive recovery and restoration, so that the observer can understand environmental properties that reduce mental fatigue and stress **Figures 1** and 2 [57].

Since Gesler introduced the concept in 1992, the notion of "therapeutic landscape" has been productively employed to better understand the dynamic between place and wellness [58], a therapeutic landscape includes both the

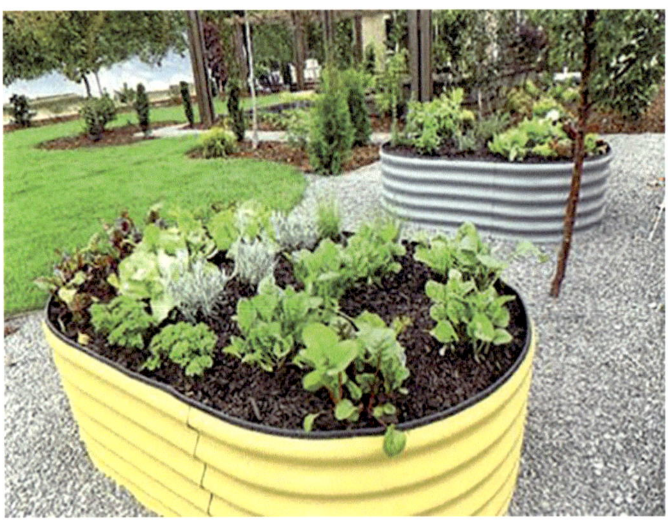

Figure 1.
Low-cost, edible garden interventions in a public park can be added as a temporary or permanent feature [57].

natural, built, symbolic, and social environments [59]. Moving from its initial application of understanding places reputed for their healing qualities, the therapeutic landscape concept today also encompasses everyday landscapes [60]. Collectively, therapeutic places are culturally constructed, experienced differently by different people, and not necessarily ideal or romantic landscapes [61]. As Gesler and Kearns [62] contend, landscapes are multi-dimensional: the sites of human-environment interaction, products of social processes, and individual or personal constructs. Similarly, contemporary definitions of health include multiple aspects of wellbeing: emotional, spiritual, physical, and social. Gesler's concept suggests that specific landscapes not only provide an identity, satisfying a human need for roots, but can also act as the location of social networks, providing settings for therapeutic activities. This is based on an understanding of the ways in which environmental, societal, and individual factors can work together to preserve health and well-being. Hence, place is understood as being relational, influenced not only by the physical environment, but also by the human mind and material circumstances—reflecting both human agency (through intentions and actions) as well as the structures and constraints imposed by society [63]. Stress, a complex, documentary, and very important

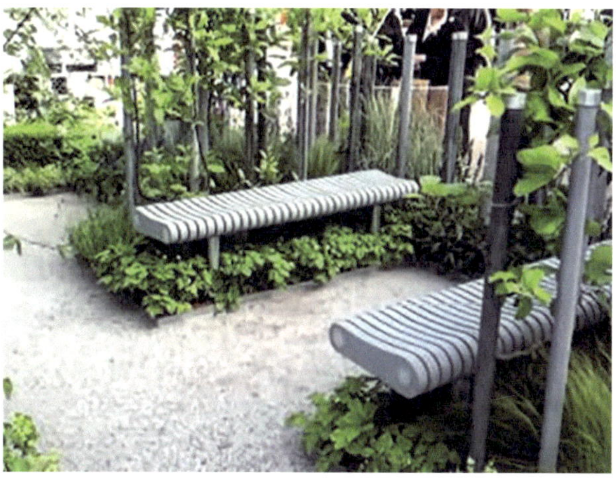

Figure 2.
London: a calm, communal public space, with edible planting, in a therapeutic garden for people living with post-traumatic stress [57].

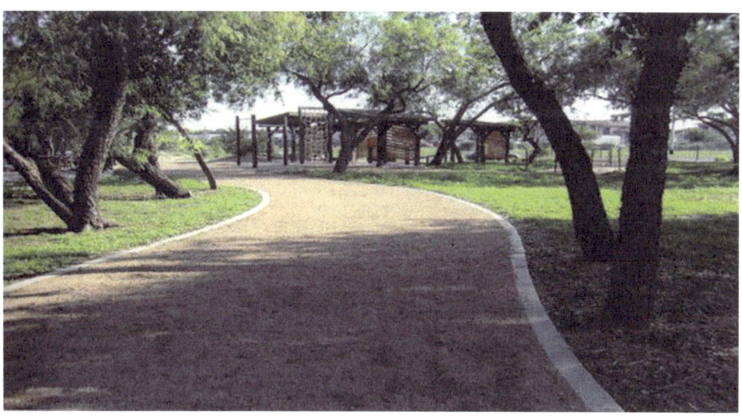

Figure 3.
PT-guided: performance physical Therapy's "PT guided fitness program" [57].

health issue, points to the importance of the issue of natural regeneration as a key advantage for PTSD to use for healing therapeutics.

According to above, one of the best ways to avoid tension from patient with PTSD treatment is to take refuge in nature. Studies have shown that the presence of plants in the environment reduces blood pressure, heart rate, muscle tension, stress, fatigue, and aggressive behavior, and factors such as level of comfort, tolerance and self-esteem, sense of well-being, life expectancy and enjoy the work environment. As defined by the World Health Organization (WHO), health is a physical, psychological, and social well-being, not just a lack of illness or illness, so the therapeutic landscape is a setting whose maximum design is trying to create healing properties in space. In fact, healing gardens through connection through human senses can heal and reduce the stress of everyday life. Evidences show that the following factors are effective in reducing stress in such spaces: good feelings from the nature, exercise and activity, social support, sense of control **Figure 3**.

5. Conclusion

Based on the above sections , in **Table 1** provides indicators status in a therapeutic landscape for people with PTSD.

How impact on health	Indicators status in a therapeutic landscape for people with PTSD	Therapeutic landscape Indicators
Stress reduction	Not too open and not too close	Balance between open and enclosed spaces
Reduced illness/positive distraction	Planting diversity, the use of short and long plants in combination with the use of green, blue and colorful landscapes	Vegetable diversity
Reducing stress and anxiety	Flexibility in various scales and elements such as paths, furniture activities, etc.	Flexibility
Reducing stress/decreasing blood pressure/decreasing anger	Abstraction and complexity for patients who are stressed are unacceptable	Minimizing ambiguity
Reducing stress/making sense of security for more mobility	Providing road safety for patients with mobility problems [slope, stairs, floors], proper lighting for the area	Create a sense of security
Reduce stress and calm down	The bird's attraction, the sound of the wind flow among the foliage, the sound of water	Decrease undesirable environmental noise and increase natural sounds
Positive distraction/stress reduction	The limited presence of some animals in some spaces [for example, the presence of fish in a pond or domestic birds]	Create a small ecosystem
Reduced heart rate/reduced anger/concentration	Use of water in ponds, lakes, etc.	Proper use of water
Positive effect on memory and navigation/decreased heart rate and blood pressure/decreased depression	Flora and plant species diversity, fruit trees	Spread flowers and plants of colorful and fragrant

How impact on health	Indicators status in a therapeutic landscape for people with PTSD	Therapeutic landscape Indicators
Reduce anger and depression/improve general state/increase cognitive capacity	Creating ground-level pots suitable for people with PTSD with physical restrictions [like wheelchairs]	Creating a workplace for horticulture
Reduce stress/decrease depression/ improve memory, concentration and senses	The presence of attractive elements along the way to increase motivation and proper flooring, as well as the creation of shadows is essential	Create spaces for strolling

Table 1.
Conclusion.

Author details

Shima Taheri[1]*, Amirhosein Shabani[2] and Maryam Ghasemi Sichani[3]

1 Young Researchers and Elite Club, Islamic Azad University, Isfahan (Khorasgan) Branch, Isfahan, Iran

2 Department of Urban Planning, Islamic Azad University, Najafabad Branch, Najafabad, Iran

3 Architecture Department, Faculty of Architecture and Urban Planning, Islamic Azad University of Isfahan (Khorasgan) Branch, Isfahan, Iran

*Address all correspondence to: shimataheri@rocketmail.com

References

[1] Smeltzer SC, Brenda G. Brunner and Suddrath's Text Book of Medical Surgical Nursing. 10th ed. Philadelphia: Lippincott; 2002

[2] Ann Sloan D. Environmental Psychology and Human Well-Being Effects of Built and Natural Settings. Cambridge: Academic Press; 2018, 482 p

[3] Compeanab E. Hamnerab: Posttraumatic stress disorder with secondary psychotic features (PTSD-SP): Diagnostic and treatment challenges. Progress in Neuro-Psychopharmacology and Biological Psychiatry. 2019;**88**:265-275

[4] Naderi Y, Moradi AR, Hasani J, Noohi S. Effectiveness of emotional schema therapy on cognitive emotion regulation strategies of combat-related post traumatic stress disorder veterans. Iranian Journal of War and Public Health. 2015;**7**(3):147-155

[5] Shalev AY, Yehuda R, McFarlane AC. International Handbook of Human Response to Trauma. New York: Kluwer Academic/Plenum Press; 2000

[6] Cooper Marcus C, Naomi S. Therapeutic Landscapes: An Evidence Based Approach to Designing Healing Gardens and Restorative Outdoor Spaces. New York :John Wiley & Sons Inc; 2014

[7] US Department of Veterans Affairs. PTSD: National Center for PTSD [Internet]. 2016. Available from: http://www.ptsd.va.gov/professional/PTSD-overview/index.asp [Accessed: 07 April 2016]

[8] Campbell DG, Felker BL, Liu C-F, Yano EM, Kirchner JE, Chan D, et al. Prevalence of depression–PTSD comorbidity: Implications for clinical practice guidelines and primary care-based interventions. Journal of General Internal Medicine. 2007;**22**(6):711-810

[9] Ginzburg K, Ein-Dor T, Solomon Z. Comorbidity of posttraumatic stress disorder, anxiety and depression: A 20-year longitudinal study of war veterans. Journal of Affective Disorders. 2010;**123**(1):249-257

[10] Breslau N, Davis GC, Schultz LR. Posttraumatic stress disorder and the incidence of nicotine, alcohol, and other drug disorders in persons who have experienced trauma. Archives of General Psychiatry. 2003;**60**(3):289-294

[11] Jakupcak M, Cook J, Imel Z, Fontana A, Rosenheck R, McFall M. Posttraumatic stress disorder as a risk factor for suicidal ideation in Iraq and Afghanistan war veterans. Journal of Traumatic Stress. 2009;**22**(4):303-306

[12] Goodnight J, Ragsdale K, Sam R, Rothbaum BO. Psychotherapy for PTSD: An evidence-based guide to a theranostic approach to treatment. Progress in Neuro-psychopharmacology Biological Psychiatry. 2019;**10**(88):418-426

[13] Purtle J. Heroes' invisible wounds of war: Constructions of posttraumatic stress disorder in the text of US federal legislation. Social Science & Medicine. 2016;**149**:9-16

[14] Prigerson HG, Maciejewski PK, Rosenheck RA. Population attributable fractions of psychiatric disorders and behavioral outcomes associated with combat exposure among US men. American Journal of Public Health. 2002;**92**(1):59-63

[15] Kessler RC, Chiu W, Demler O, Walters EE, Revalence P. Severity, and comorbidity of 12-month DSM-IV disorders in the national comorbidity survey replication. Archives of General Psychiatry. 2005;**62**(6):617-627

[16] Hatzenbuehler ML, Phelan JC, Link BG. Stigma as a fundamental cause of population health inequalities. American Journal of Public Health. 2013;**103**(5):813-821

[17] Ghaffarzadegan N, Ebrahimvandi A, Jalali MS. A dynamic model of post-traumatic stress disorder for military personnel and veterans. PLoS ONE. 2016;**11**(10):e0161405

[18] Ahmadizadeh M, Khodabakh A, Jafar A. The effectiveness of problem solving and prolonged exposure therapy methods and a combination of both on the adjustment of veterans suffering from war-related post-traumatic stress disorder. Journal of Military Medicine. 2012;**14**(3):178-185

[19] Noohi AM, Tavallaei SA, Karami GR. Post-traumatic stress disorder (PTSD) among aggressive patients attending to Baqiyatallah psychiatric clinic in 2005. Journal of Military Medicine. 2006;**8**(3):175-181

[20] Davidson J. Trauma: The impact of posttraumatic stress disorder. Journal of Psychopharmacology. 2000;**14**(2):S5-S12

[21] Cao H, McFarlane AC, Klimidis S. Prevalence of psychiatric disorder following the 1988 Yun Nan (China) earthquake. Social Psychiatry and Psychiatric Epidemiology. 2003;**38**(4):204-212

[22] Galea S, Vlahov D, Resnick H, Ahern J, Susser E, Gold J. Trends of probable post-traumatic stress disorder in New York City after the September 11 terrorist attacks. American Journal of Epidemiology. 2003;**158**(6):514-524

[23] Parandeh A, Khaghanizadeh M, Karimi Zarchi A. The effect of training conflict resolution on quality of life's on spouses of war veterans post traumatic stress disorder. Journal of Military Medicine. 2006;**8**(1):45-51

[24] Halligan SL, Yehuda R. Risk factors for PTSD. PTSD Research Quarterly. 2000;**11**(3):1-3

[25] Kozaric-Kovacic D, Kocijan-Hercigonja D. Assessment of post-traumatic stress disorder and comorbidity. Military Medicine. 2001;**166**(8):677-680

[26] Kozaric-Kovacic D, Kocijan-Hercigonja D, Grubisic-Ilic M. Posttraumatic stress disorder and depression in soldiers with combat experiences. Croatian Medical Journal. 2001;**42**(2):165-170

[27] Sharma S, Ressler KJ. Genomic updates in understanding PTSD. Progress in Neuro-Psychopharmacology and Biological Psychiatry. 2019;**90**:197-203

[28] Korpela K, Hartig T. Restorative qualities of favorite places. Journal of Environmental Psychology. 1996;**16**:221-233

[29] Mitchell R, Popham F. Green space, urbanity and health: Relationships in England. Journal of Epidemiology and Community Health. 2007;**61**:681-683

[30] Richardson E, Mitchell R. Gender differences in relationships between urban green space and health in the United Kingdom. Social Science & Medicine. 2010;**71**(3):568-575

[31] Mitchell R, Pearce J, Shortt N. Place, space and health inequalities. In: Smith K, Bambra C, Hill S, editors. Health Inequalities: Critical Perspectives. Oxford: OUP; 2015

[32] Kaplan S. The restorative benefits of nature: Toward an integrative framework. Journal of Environmental Psychology. 1995;**15**(31):69-182

[33] Kaplan R, Kaplan S. Adolescents and the natural environment: A time out? In: Kahn PH Jr, Kellert SR, editors. Children

and Nature: Theoretical, Conceptual, and Empirical Investigations. Cambridge, MA: MIT Press; 2002

[34] Pretty J, Peacock J, Sellens M, Griffin M. The mental and physical health outcomes of green exercise. International Journal of Environmental Health Research. 2005;**15**:319-337

[35] Hartig T. Issues in restorative environments research: Matters of measurement. In: Fernández B, Hidalgo C, Salvador C, Martos MJ, editors. Psicología Ambiental: Entre los Estudios Urbanos y el análisis de la Sostenibilidad. Almería: PSICAMB; 2011

[36] Kuo FE, Taylor AF. The potential natural treatment for attention deficit/hyperactivity disorder: Evidence for a national study. American Journal of Public Health. 2004;**94**:1580-1586

[37] Moore M, Townsend M, Oldroyd J. Linking human and ecosystem health: The benefits of community involvement in conservation groups. EcoHealth. 2006;**3**:255-261

[38] Maller C, Townsend M, Pryor A, Brown P, St Leger L. Healthy nature healthy people: 'Contact with nature' as an upstream health promotion intervention for populations. Health Promotion International. 2006;**21**(1):45-54

[39] Ulrich R. View through a window may influence recovery from surgery. Science Journal. 1984;**224**(4647):420-421

[40] Kofler W. Ecology and Forests for Public Health. Munich: International Council for Scientific Development; 2010

[41] Marberry SO. A Conversation with Roger Ulrich. Healthcare Design. 2010. Available from: www.healthcaredesignmagazine.com/article/conversation-rogerUlrich?Page=show [Accessed: 01 November 2010]

[42] Taheri S, Shabani A. Conceptual and practical principles in designing healing gardens for veterans with PTSD with a focus on reducing stress—A narrative review. Journal of Molecular Medicine. 2016;**18**(3):230-241

[43] Hartig T, Evans G, Jamner LD, Davis DS, Garling T. Tracking restoration in natural and urban field settings. Journal of Environmental Psychology. 2003;**23**:109-123

[44] Ulrich R. Effects of gardens on health outcomes: Theory and research. In: Cooper Marcus C, Barnes M, editors. Healing Gardens: Therapeutic Benefits and Design Recommendations. New York: John Wiley; 1991

[45] Berto R. The role of nature in coping with psycho-physiological stress: A literature review on restorativeness. Behavioral Sciences (Basel). 2014;**4**(4):394-409

[46] Sachs NA. Interview with Dr. Esther Sternberg, Author of Healing Spaces: The Science of Place and Well-Being [Internet]. 2009. Available from: www.healinglandscape.org/blog/2009/09/interview-with-dr-esthersternberg-author-of-healing-spaces-the-science-of-the-place-and-well-being [Accessed: 01 September 2009]

[47] Sternberg EM. Healing Spaces: The Science and Place of Well-Being. Cambridge, MA: Harvard University Press; 2010

[48] Kuo FE, Sullivan WC. Environment and crime in the inner city: Does vegetation reduce crime? Environment and Behavior. 2001;**33**(3):343-367

[49] Kuo FE. Coping with poverty: Impacts of environment and attention in the inner city. Environment and Behavior. 2001;**33**(1):5-34

[50] Kuo FE, Sullivan WC. Aggression and violence in the inner city: Impacts of environment via mental fatigue. Environment and Behavior. 2001;**33**(4):543-571

[51] Li Q, Morimoto K, Nakadai A, Inagaki H, Katsumata M, Shimizu T, et al. Forest bathing enhances human natural killer activity and expression of anti-cancer proteins. International Journal of Immunopathology and Pharmacology. 2007;**20**:3-8

[52] Lindemuth AL. Greening in the Red Zone: Disaster, Resilience, and Community Greening. Netherland: Springer; 2014

[53] Francis C, Cooper Marcus C. Places people take their problems. In: Proceedings of Annual Conference of Environmental Design and Research Association. 1991;**22**:178-84

[54] Ulrich R. Effects of healthcare environmental design on medical outcomes design and health. In: Proceedings Design and Health World Congress and Exhibition; Stockholm: 2001. pp. 49-69

[55] Ulrich R. Health Benefits of Gardens in Hospitals. Paper for conference, Plants for People International Exhibition Florida; 2002

[56] Kaplan R, Kaplan S. The Experience of Nature: A Psychological Perspective. Cambridge: Cambridge University Press; 1989

[57] Souter-Brown G. Landscape and Urban Design for Health and Well-Being: Using Healing, Sensory and Therapeutic Gardens. London:Routledge Press; 2015

[58] Williams A. Therapeutic Landscapes: The Dynamic between Place and Wellness. Lanham, MD: University Press of America; 1999. pp. 1-11

[59] Baer LD, Gesler WM. Reconsidering the concept of therapeutic landscapes in JD Salinger's the Catcherin the Rye. Area. 2004;**36**(4):404-413

[60] Thorsen RS. Conceptualizations of pluralistic medical fields: Exploring the therapeutic landscapes of Nepal. Health and Place. 2014;**31**:83-89

[61] Dunkley CM. A therapeutic taskscape: Theorizing place-making, discipline and care at a camp for troubled youth. Health and Place. 2008;**15**:88-96

[62] Gesler W, Kearns RA. Culture/Place/Health. London and New York: Routledge; 2002

[63] Milligan C. 'Cultivating health': Therapeutic landscapes and older people in northern England. Social Science and Medicine. 2004;**58**:1781-1793

Chapter 7

Videoconferencing Psychotherapy in an App Environment for Trauma-Related Psychopathology

Annemiek van Dijke and Jacques van Lankveld

Abstract

The theoretical background of the life-span sequelae of exposure to interpersonal psychological trauma (emotional or physical neglect or abuse or sexual abuse) in childhood, particularly when a primary caretaker is involved, and its assessment and treatment possibilities in a 100% online environment are outlined. These sequelae may be understood as a complex variant of PTSD (CPTSD) or a complicated array of overlapping mental and personality disorders or as trans-diagnostic symptoms. However, disorders of extreme stress not otherwise specified (DESNOS) constitute a distinct syndrome of potential clinical utility. In childhood, adolescence, and young adulthood (YA), these symptoms seem encompassed by developmental trauma disorder (DTD). Affect dysregulation, identity alterations, and relational impairment are central features of DESNOS/DTD/CPTSD and can also be understood as trans-diagnostic symptom clusters. More and more people use smartphone apps in daily life. Therefore we started our 100% online treatments in patients' environments and at their convenience (need driven). Our digitally enriched outpatient clinics (DOCs) using smartphone apps for videoconferencing psychotherapy (VCP) and personal data monitoring aim to augment established evidence-based treatment protocols. Also, they facilitate continuously gathering real-time sensor- and self-reported data that improve ecological validity of self-reports and monitoring for course of treatment and relapse prevention.

Keywords: childhood trauma, smartphone, app, videoconferencing psychotherapy, PTSD

1. Introduction

1.1 The life-span sequelae of exposure to interpersonal psychological trauma (emotional or physical neglect or abuse or sexual abuse) in childhood

Caretaker-related traumatic stressors are likely to occur in and contribute to a relational growth-inhibiting early environment, interfere with the development of optimal set points and strive for homeostasis of basic brain functioning, and may therefore adversely impact the development of self- and affect regulation capacities in childhood. Infants of caretakers who are unresponsive or poorly affectively attuned are at risk for developing insecure attachment. Infants who additionally experience an abusive caretaker are at risk for developing post-traumatic states of

IntechOpen

enduring negative affect that may become disorganized attachment working models and chronic dysfunctional self- and affect regulation patterns. Such sequelae of early life "neurodevelopmental injuries" have been described as epidemic and understudied [1].

Also, the life-span sequelae of exposure to interpersonal psychological trauma (emotional or physical neglect or abuse or sexual abuse) in childhood, particularly when a primary caretaker is involved, do not seem to be encompassed by any single DSM disorder [2]. Symptoms include and extend symptoms associated with post-traumatic stress disorder (PTSD) with and without dissociative symptoms. Also, it has been argued that these sequelae also include a complex symptom presentation reflecting disturbances in (interpersonal) self-regulatory capacities and mental disorders that may occur comorbidly with or separately from PTSD [3]. Whether these sequelae are best understood as a complex variant of PTSD (CPTSD) or a complicated array of overlapping mental and personality disorders is controversial [4, 5]. However, there is mounting evidence that a disorder of extreme stress not otherwise specified (DESNOS) formulation of CPTSD constitutes a distinct syndrome of potential clinical utility [6, 7]. In childhood, adolescence, and young adulthood (YA), these symptoms seem encompassed by the developmental trauma disorder (DTD) formulation [8].

1.2 Affect dysregulation, identity alterations, and relational impairment

Three core features of the DESNOS formulation of CPTSD symptomatology and DTD were identified based on a comprehensive literature review [8]: affect dysregulation, identity alterations (dissociation), and relational impairment (insecure attachment) [3, 9–12].

Affect dysregulation is defined as problems in experiencing, managing (keeping emotional arousal within the Window of Tolerance (WoT) [13]), or recovering from extreme states of affect, including both under-regulation of heightened affect states and maladaptive overregulation of affect (e.g., [14]). Under-regulation involves limited access to or capacity for deploying strategies to reduce intense affect states and associated difficulties with impulse control and goal-directed behavior (e.g., anger that escalates into rage or anxiety that becomes an unmanageable state of terror). Overregulation involves nonacceptance and limited awareness or clarity of emotions (e.g., states of profound emotional emptiness or detachment) [15]. The latter has also been defined as alexithymia [16]. Alexithymia type I is characterized by low emotionality and a poor fantasy life in combination with poorly developed cognitions accompanying the emotions. This type is also referred to as core or full-blown alexithymia and displays both cognitive and affective alexithymia (e.g., [17, 18]). Alexithymia type II only suffers from cognitive alexithymia and is characterized by high emotionality and a rich fantasy life in combination with poorly developed cognitions accompanying the emotions. Alexithymia type II has been associated with childhood sexual abuse and PTSD symptoms (e.g., [19]).

Clinically, Lane differentiated levels of emotional awareness (LEAS; e.g., [20]), a three-dimensional cognitive-developmental framework that LEAS scores plausibly track, including the transition from focusing on external/physical to internal/psychological characteristics, greater conceptual complexity, and self-other differentiation. This concept is closely related to differentiating alexithymia types but highlights the cognitive-developmental character of emotional maturation and also taps into affective agnosia.

Identity alterations involve problems with maintaining a coherent sense of (mental and embodied) self within the WoT, which may take the form of dissociation symptoms including somatoform or embodied dissociative symptoms such as conversion symptoms, pain, or somatization and psychoform or mentalized dissociative symptoms such as depersonalization, amnesia, or identity alterations that may turn into positive or negative forms of dissociation (e.g., [15, 21]). Trauma-related overwhelming affect and its dysfunctional regulation compromise the integrative capacities associated with cognitive-emotional information processing so that information becomes disassociated, disorganized, or disoriented (e.g., [22]). Janet [23] introduced his model of the mind consisting of two different ways of functioning: (a) activities that preserve and reproduce the past and (b) activities which are directed toward synthesis and creation (i.e., integration). In line with Janet, Van der Hart and colleagues consider dissociation a core feature of trauma: a division of personality into dissociative (biopsychosocial) subsystems that evolve when the individual lacks the capacity to integrate adverse experiences in part or in full, as can be recognized in dissociative identity disorder (DID) patients [23]. Already in Janet's original research (and recently further conceptualized), the existence of dissociative subsystems manifests in positive and negative dissociative symptoms (e.g., dissociative flashback episodes; e.g., in [23]). These positive and negative dissociative symptoms can be further distinguished as psychoform and somatoform dissociative symptoms (e.g., [24]). Negative dissociative symptoms refer to apparent losses of functions, for example, of memory, motor control, skills, and somatosensory awareness. Negative psychoform dissociative symptoms, among others, include loss of memory (amnesia) and loss of affective experiencing (numbness), loss of needs and will (abulia), loss of critical function (a cognitive action) resulting in suggestibility and difficulty thinking things through, loss of previously existing skills, and diminished sense of self. Negative somatoform dissociative symptoms, among others, involve loss of sensory-perceptual or motor functions, e.g., analgesia, paralysis, and aphonia. Positive psychoform dissociative symptoms include traumatic memories and nightmares that have affective, cognitive, and somatosensory components such as dissociative flashbacks and full re-experiencing of traumatizing events, as well as intruding voices, thoughts, and amplified affective experiencing. Positive somatoform dissociative symptoms include intrusions of sensorimotor aspects of traumatic re-experiences, including pain, uncontrolled behaviors such as tics, sensory distortions, and pseudo-epileptic seizures.

Relational impairment in adulthood involves two dimensions [25] that have been shown to have better internal consistency than the prototypical secure, preoccupied, dismissing, and unresolved attachment categories and to provide a good fit in confirmatory factor analyses: avoidance (i.e., fear of closeness) and anxiety (i.e., fear of abandonment) [26]. Attachment-related avoidance and anxiety were selected to represent adult relational impairment rather than the childhood-based categories of insecure attachment because they were shown to be trait-like risk factors for self-reported psychiatric symptoms (i.e., correlated with psychopathology under conditions of both high and low stress), while the insecure attachment categories were associated with psychopathology in adults only under high-stress conditions [27]. When confronted with potential threatening events, the primary attachment strategy (secure attachment) involves proximity seeking: attempting to move closer, physically or emotionally or both, to persons who are perceived as providing relational security that can serve to alleviate distress and build or access resources, remaining within the WoT. When external (real) or internalized (i.e., working model representations of) attachment figures are unavailable, secondary attachment strategies (insecure attachment: hyper-activation or deactivation of the internalized attachment system) are hypothesized to be activated in order to cope with relational insecurity and related distress: failure of remaining within the WoT. Secondary attachment strategies involve a defensive focus either on fear of abandonment (i.e., attempts to restore proximity and reduce anxiety; hence hyper-activation) or fear of closeness (i.e., attempts to inhibit proximity seeking and reduce awareness of distress; hence deactivation/inhibition). Clinically and phenomenologically, the secondary attachment strategies appear to involve relatively distinct forms of emotion dysregulation, with under-regulation of emotion predominating in fear of abandonment and overregulation of emotion characterizing fear of closeness [25].

Overall, dysfunctional self-regulation is the core of these problems.

1.3 Childhood interpersonal trauma-related disorders

Although the life-span sequelae of exposure to psychological trauma-by-primary-caretaker in childhood do not seem to be encompassed by any single DSM disorder [2], the DESNOS formulation of CPTSD in adulthood and DTD in adolescence-YA has been demonstrated *empirically* to be associated with childhood relational adverse experiences that are potentially traumatic (e.g., maltreatment, family violence) consistently across numerous studies [10–12, 28, 29].

CPTSD as defined by DESNOS is theorized to represent the results of developmental adaptations to exposure to interpersonal trauma in developmentally sensitive periods, including altered emotion processing, dissociative shifts in self-awareness and consciousness, and disruption of secure attachment working models (e.g., see [7]).

Borderline personality disorder (BPD) arguably involves similar forms of dysregulation, and, historically, symptoms of somatic symptom disorders (SSD) have been associated with interpersonal trauma and hysteria [6]. Nevertheless, CPTSD can be distinguished in terms of clinical phenomenology from PTSD, BPD, SSD, anxiety disorders, and depression. CPTSD as defined by DESNOS appears to involve hypervigilance related to being harmed, whereas BPD involves extreme sensitivity to perceiving oneself as being abandoned or rejected/shamed [6, 30].

Moreover, certain features of CPTSD that are conceptually related to PTSD (i.e., arousal-related somatic dysregulation; altered personal schemas) may be largely accounted for by PTSD, but CPTSD features that are more clinically and conceptually distinct from PTSD (i.e., affect dysregulation, dissociation) appear to be empirically distinct from PTSD in adults with severe psychopathology [30].

1.4 Network theory of trauma

As opposed to trying to categorize symptoms within existing classifications/diagnoses (e.g., dissociative subtype of PTSD), or attempting to get new diagnoses accepted (e.g., DESNOS, CPTSD, DTD), the life-span sequelae of exposure to interpersonal psychological trauma (emotional or physical neglect or abuse or sexual abuse) in childhood can also be understood as *trans-diagnostic* phenomenology.

Network theory supports this trans-diagnostic perspective. According to Borsboom (e.g., [31]), the comprehensive theoretical model of (trauma-related) psychopathology follows five principles to encode the backbone of the *network theory* of mental disorders:

Principle 1. Complexity: Mental disorders are best characterized in terms of the interaction between different components in a psychopathology network.

Principle 2. Symptom-component correspondence: The components in the psychopathology network correspond to the problems that have been codified as symptoms in the past century and appear as such in current diagnostic manuals.

Principle 3. Direct causal connections: The network structure is generated by a pattern of direct causal connections between symptoms.

Principle 4. Mental disorders follow network structure: The psychopathology network has a nontrivial topology, in which certain symptoms are more tightly connected than others. These symptom groupings give rise to the phenomenological manifestation of mental disorders as groups of symptoms that often arise together.

These principles imply that the etiology of mental disorders can be thought of in terms of a process of spreading activation in a symptom network. If a symptom arises (which may occur for different reasons depending on person, time, and context), this will increase the probability that a connected symptom arises as well. Thus, coupled sets of symptoms, which are close in the network structure, will tend to synchronize. Mental disorders then arise when groups of tightly coupled symptoms actively maintain each other, leading to a cluster of psychopathology symptoms that becomes self-sustaining [31].

Principle 5. Hysteresis: Mental disorders arise due to the presence of hysteresis in strongly connected symptom networks: the network can become self-sustaining, which implies that *symptoms continue to activate each other, even after the triggering cause of the disorder has disappeared*. Although the presence of a trigger can activate a strong network, *the absence/disappearance of that trigger does not deactivate the strongly connected network*. This may well be the explanation for PTSD symptoms and attachment trauma-related insecure self-regulation styles, which develop and endure after the traumatic events have subsided as observed in attachment-trauma patients (DESNOS/DTD).

1.5 Inhibitory, excitatory, and combined inhibitory and excitatory (IE) regulation

Despite a vast amount of research on the benefits of successfully regulating affect for our mental well-being, the role of dysfunctional self- and affect regulation for psychiatric patients remains unclear. However, it has been established that affect dysregulation is involved in the etiology of psychopathology and that dysfunctional self-regulation is often described in patients with complex psychopathology and mental disorders. Dysfunctional affect regulation typically seems to involve an interpersonal context, and attachment theory has become a prominent conceptual framework for understanding the process of development of affect regulation and dysregulation. Whereas some patients react to adversities with inhibited experiencing and social withdrawal, others react hyper-emotionally and tend to cling to a significant other to alleviate (interpersonal) stress and regulate to baseline and return within the WoT.

The DESNOS formulation of CPTSD in adulthood and developmental trauma disorder (DTD) in childhood and adolescence have been demonstrated empirically to be associated with qualitatively different self-regulation strategies/styles or three different networks: inhibitory, excitatory, and combined inhibitory and excitatory (IE) regulation (see **Figure 1**; e.g., [7]). Symptoms include disturbances in self-regulation across several domains of functioning, including affective-, cognitive-, somatic-, relational-, reflective-, executive-, behavioral-, and psycho-physiological functioning. Activation of dysfunctional regulation seems to follow trauma-by-primary-caretaker associated negatively biased cognitive-emotional information processing. However, when potentially neutral situations are processed and evaluated as threatening or potentially harmful, dysfunctional regulation is activated false positively. Consequently, this may result in interpersonal misunderstanding and disappointments, which in turn condition and uphold the insecure attachment representation/working models eventually turning into dysfunctional regulation vicious circles.

Mental states associated with *inhibited experiencing* are consistent with overregulation of affect and with the negative psychoform and somatoform dissociative symptoms, including appearing emotionally constricted, expressionless, machine-like, weak or frozen, social avoidant, rigid mental elaborations or mental blancs,

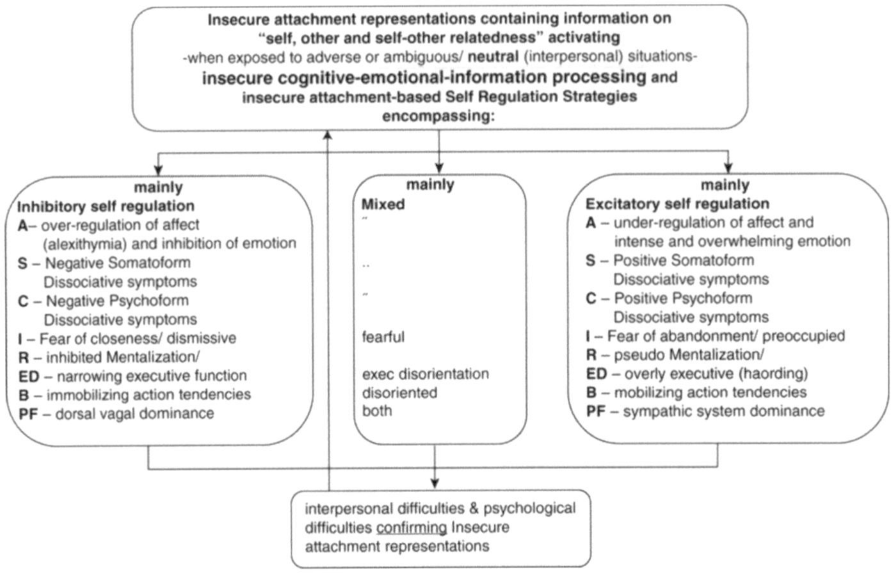

Figure 1.
Three qualitatively different self-regulation styles or different networks: inhibitory, excitatory, and combined inhibitory and excitatory (IE) regulation operating in self-sustaining, vicious cycles due to the presence of hysteresis in strongly connected childhood trauma-related symptom networks.

diminished reflective functioning, low or cramped nerve, muscle tension, etc. Mental states associated with *excitatory experiencing* are consistent with under-regulation of affect and with the positive psychoform and somatoform dissociative symptoms, including feeling overwhelmed, seizures, hyper-alertness, impulsivity, and difficulty handling intense emotion states. Mental states associated with *combined or altering inhibited and excitatory experiencing* present clinically with mixed features of inhibitory and excitatory (IE) regulation and are associated with more complex psychopathology and DESNOS/DTD (see **Figure 1**; e.g., see [7]).

1.6 Basic affective systems in the brain and trauma

Panksepp and Biven argue that the basic brain functions strive for survival and homeostasis [32]. Seven basic affective-motivational systems are differentiated, located deep in the most ancient, subcortical regions of mammalian brains: SEEKING (expectancy), FEAR (anxiety), RAGE (anger), LUST (sexual excitement), CARE (nurturance), PANIC/GRIEF (sadness), and PLAY (social joy). Affects need no higher cognitive brain function to work appropriately, nor do they need the ability to use words to express themselves. They are the rawest form of emotional experiencing. In fact, these are referred to as the primary-process emotions. The theory of a SEEKING system has been studied for decades. It stems from the research done on the brain reward system, but it attempts to explain behaviors beyond a simple motivation for a reward. It is not just the reward itself that pushes one to learn, but it is the whole process of reinforcement that urges one to learn new things. "This general-purpose SEEKING response not only helps [animals] spontaneously look for and, with luck and skill, find the resources that they need, but also the means of escaping from danger, which they eventually need to learn to avoid. All this entails looking around and exploring the environment" (p. 133). Individuals can experience problems when something is amiss with the SEEKING system. FEAR systems were designed to help anticipate bad things in the future, and through the process of experience, they become capable of anticipating bad things. FEAR, like every other emotional system, is born essentially "objectless," and, like all other emotional systems of the BrainMind, it becomes connected to the real world through learning. FEAR produces terror and promotes chronic anxiety in response to milder, more sustained arousal. However, this system can also become sensitized and overactive, especially if it has been repeatedly traumatized, as is the case in PTSD and other trauma-related disorders [32]. Overactivation and sensitization of the PANIC/GRIEF (sadness) system can be recognized in our patients reporting disrupted attachment bonds or severe emotional neglect, a different kind of traumatization.

However, conditions arising from an overstimulated FEAR or PANIC/GRIEF system, such as chronic anxiety, can be treated through a process of learning. The mind is capable of reconsolidating memories, a phenomenon useful for psychotherapy. By retrieving memories in a different affective context, it can soften the feelings of negative memories. It is their hope that, "Fearful memories can be erased or overridden by 'therapeutic' maneuvers that cleverly use the consolidation process against itself" (p. 208). The CARE system is intertwined with the SEEKING system. The CARE system is at work in the therapist/patient relationship. "Effective psychotherapists share their ability for CARE, along with the ability to recruit the healing power of positive emotions" (p. 310) [32]. Especially in attachment-trauma cases, we can recognize these seven basic affective systems, with disturbed functioning in complex PTSD. Too much FEAR, RAGE, and PANIC/GRIEF and too little SEEKING, CARE, and PLAY are often recognized in our patients.

The therapist and the therapeutic relationship therefore facilitate and promote learning in a secure and attuned stimulating environment.

1.7 Bad lifestyle, risk behavior, ill health, and physical illness in relation to trauma

Dysfunctional self- and affect regulation, sensitization, and overactivation of FEAR, RAGE, and PANIC/GRIEF systems may result in bad lifestyle, risk behavior, ill health, and physical illness. Bad lifestyle, risk behavior, ill health, and physical illness have also been associated with exposure to interpersonal psychological trauma (emotional or physical neglect or abuse or sexual abuse) in childhood (many publications, e.g., [33, 34]). The ACE studies by Kaiser Permanente revealed the vast prevalence of physical illness and early death in childhood trauma survivors [33]. Others found the presence of ill health as well as health-undermining behavior to be overrepresented in patients reporting childhood traumas [33, 34]. Difficulties with self- and affect regulation are related to bad lifestyle and risk behavior. Also, the overactivation of insecure attachment-based self-dysregulation strategies may burden organs, e.g., the heart, and stress hormone-releasing activity to the extent of function failure and physical illness.

2. Digitally enriched outpatient clinics (DOCs) using smartphone app for videoconferencing psychotherapy (VCP) and personal data monitoring

2.1 Use of smartphones

People are becoming more and more supported by technology, and many people use smartphones with apps. Therefore we initiated digitally enriched outpatient clinics using a smartphone app for videoconferencing psychotherapy and ecological momentary assessment (EMA) in the Netherlands. Our DOCs provide technology-supported, evidence-based treatment (including, but not limited to, cognitive-behavior therapy) in patients' environments and at their convenience in an app environment. Also, EMA facilitates continuously gathering real-time sensor- and self-reported data that improve ecological validity of the results of self-reports and outcome monitoring.

Symptoms are considered consequences of mutually reinforcing demographic, personal, social, and contextual factors and (interpersonal) life events that differ for each individual and can change over time. Assessment and monitoring happen intuitively and take place in the here and now of their social and personal contexts in an app environment, rather than discretely, retrospectively, or in an isolated static moment outside the patient's personal world, thereby enriching information relevant for course of treatment, recovery, and (relapse) prevention for similar or different illness over a longer period of time.

There is currently an urgent need for psychotherapeutic interventions that use less therapist time, with the same or better outcomes than with traditional face-to-face therapy (e.g., [35, 36]. Anxiety disorders, including PTSD and depression, are among the top 10 most costly medical conditions (e.g., [37]).

2.2 The role of learning in relapse after treatment: transfer failures and erosion of therapy gains in trauma treatment

Major problems regarding the effectiveness of psychological interventions for (trauma-related) treatment are (1) transfer failures of change processes from therapy room to target situation, e.g., home environment, and (2) relapse after intervention termination. Both problems originate mainly from context-dependent learning in psychological change processes, implying that what is learned in one context generalizes insufficiently to other (target) contexts, and that learned behavior is maintained by context-dependent cues and reinforcement.

Failure to generalize/transfer the mental health gains that clients experience in the practitioner's office in treatment to their situation in daily life is a major issue in mental health care. For example, in the treatment of clients with anxiety disorders, repeated exposure to the feared stimuli reliably leads to extinction of the anxiety and the disinhibition of previously learned avoidance behavior. However, confrontation with the feared stimuli in another context than the one in which exposure took place has been found to lead to reinstatement of the problematic fearful apprehension and avoidance behavior in several experimental studies as well as in comparative clinical studies [38–40]. Another major issue in the clinical practice of mental health care is relapse, referring to the recurrence of mental health problems after the termination of psychological interventions [41]. Context-specific learning processes that lead to reinstatement of fearful behavior contribute to relapse after cognitive-behavioral exposure treatment of anxiety disorders [42, 43].

Our DOCs were initiated to accommodate patients' needs with regard to modern therapy modes and overcome problems with effectiveness of psychological interventions and relapse: we aim to augment the effectiveness of existing and evidence-based psychological interventions for prevalent mental disorders, transcending transfer failure, and relapse issues. A set of ecological momentary assessment and intervention (EMAI) tools that help to facilitate transfer of psychological change to target situations helps increase the effectiveness of already existing evidence-based interventions for trauma-related disorders in home and work environments of patients. Moreover, EMAI helps to maintain these gains over time. This is pursued by incorporating the existing knowledge of well-established methods for technology-enhanced learning and contextual and cross-contextual support of learning and adapting these methods for the development of the EMAI tools in trauma-focused and trauma-informed treatment. Our DOCs build on and extend well-established, trans-diagnostic mechanisms of behavior modification and cognitive and emotional change for trauma-related (mental) health improvement. We carefully investigate the involved mechanisms of change for each patient among different types of trauma-related psychopathology. Videoconferencing technology, which allows audio and video information to be shared, is generally associated with good user satisfaction and is found to have similar clinical outcomes to traditional face-to-face psychotherapy. VCP has become well established as a feasible and acceptable mode of psychological treatment delivery.

Findings from the WHO survey reinforce the importance of (interpersonal) negative life events as a major public health problem and highlight the significance of exposure to (interpersonal) negative life events as a risk factor for mental and physical illness, learning problems, low personal and social well-being, and personal development. Learning from experience seems crucial in treatment success, resilience, and overcoming adversity. Psychotherapy is learning and facilitates learning from experience. The app will monitor the course of symptoms and function as a support tool for exercises, e.g., send reminders, prompt exposure moments, and suggest cognitive elaborations of beliefs for the therapeutic alliance. The focus of the app environment will be on overcoming dysfunctional regulation, including avoidance. Our DOCs with smartphone app environment:

1. Facilitate context-specific learning (deliver evidence-based treatment at home, work, trips, etc.).

2. Enable easy and flexible collection of personalized data (including self-report and sensor data).

3. Enable therapeutic support (VCP, chatting).

4. Enable the use of problem-solving techniques.

5. Allow for automatic, tailored, trans-diagnostic ecological momentary interventions (EMAI), based on ecological momentary assessment (EMA) of the needs and wants of clients.

6. Allow for delivery of interventions that help maintain therapy gains or prevent relapse into previous problem states based on personalized EMA and self-reports.

2.3 Therapeutic alliance

Therapeutic alliance (TA) is an essential factor underlying successful therapy across therapeutic models. A literature review overwhelmingly supported the notion that TA can be developed in psychotherapy by videoconference, with clients rating bond and presence at least equally as strongly as in-person settings across a range of diagnostic groups [44]. Therapists also rated high levels of TA, but often not quite as high as that of their clients early in treatment. The evidence was examined in the context of important aspects of TA, including bond, presence, therapist attitudes and abilities, and client attitudes and beliefs. Also, psychotherapy seems to support and enhance self-reflection. First results support the idea that patients can develop a reflective self in cyberspace [45]. VCP helps facilitate this reflective self, and our app environment embraces and mirrors the personal content using ecological momentary assessment.

Internet-based trauma-focused guided self-help for PTSD seems a promising treatment option that requires far less therapist time than current first-line face-to-face psychological therapy [46]. The Internet-based program includes eight modules that focus on psycho-education, grounding, relaxation, behavioral activation, real-life and imaginal exposure, cognitive therapy, and relapse prevention.

Our DOCs meet and extend these possibilities as our app environment includes VCP options with EMA and EMAI. Our app environment enables us to monitor and study (A) the course and effectivity of our technology-supported assessment and evidence-based treatment and (B) the course (and erosion) of therapy gains after treatment termination over a longer period of time. The premise of this model is that trauma-related symptoms and its mutual interactions differ among patients and may change over time since no one-to-one relation was found for (interpersonal) negative life events, personal characteristics, and any mental or physical illness across the life-span.

Because patients can use the app whenever they need a therapeutic intervention, treatment can be offered more flexibly and be more integrated in patients' daily life (ecological environment). The data will result in personalized information about learning in psychotherapy and potential mediators for recovery/relapse, e.g., risk profiles at treatment onset for poor treatment course/outcome, low self-esteem, interfering (covert) behavior such as risky lifestyle, positive or adverse life events, small chaotic social network, (in)secure attachment behavior, or self-transcendence that help improve assessment- and technology-supported evidence-based treatment.

After initial treatment and during follow-up, the app functions as a support tool monitoring positive and negative life events, lifestyle/somatic well-being, and interpersonal activities to detect early warning signs of potential relapse or crisis (prevention).

3. Digitally enriched therapeutic processes

3.1 Stuck in a "survival state of mind" or "historical time loop"

In our patients with complex trauma histories, we can often recognize dysfunctional self- and affect regulation: too much activity of the FEAR, RAGE, and PANIC/GRIEF systems (excitatory dysregulation; see **Figure 1**) or too little activation of the SEEKING, CARE, and PLAY systems (inhibitory dysregulation; see **Figure 1**) or a combination of both due to the presence of hysteresis.

The strongly connected symptom networks have become self-sustaining, and the absence/disappearance of the trauma-related trigger does not deactivate the network. As a result patients report in the app environment often too much negative emotional experience while undertaking few fun, relaxing, healthy, social-bonding activities. And the patient is often stuck in a "survival or destructive state of mind" or "historical time loop," thereby overruling the "learning state of mind." This may well be why complex trauma/DESNOS/DTD patients have poorer therapy outcome and quick erosion of (little to modest) therapy gains [47].

By monitoring the app content, the app possibilities facilitate the therapist to support patients when help, comfort, or encouragement is needed: hence need-driven interventions. The therapist may choose to chat with the patient or initiate a VCP session or provide the patient with useful information from the library via a link in a chat message. To help overcome the "survival or destructive state of mind" or "historical time loop," a therapist-initiated chat contact referring to a therapy motto or personal one-liner may be helpful, or a "ping" [sound] or buzz [sound + sensation] from the smartphone may help overcome depersonalization and dissociation to help the patient to transit, through realization, into a "learning or productive state of mind" associated with activation of the SEEKING, CARE, and PLAY systems and decline of excitatory and inhibitory dysregulation symptoms.

3.2 REX

For complex trauma and DESNOS/DTD, often a phase-oriented treatment program (phase 1, stabilization; phase 2, trauma therapy; and phase 3, rehabilitation) is held [48]. In the app, this was translated into the "toolbox" metaphor. During the therapy process, elements from three toolboxes (REX) are held: toolbox **R**, for self- and affect regulation techniques, healthy lifestyle, etc.; toolbox **E**, for trauma work/ exposure therapies; and toolbox **X**, for X-factor activities—fun, social activities, rehabilitation, work, and sports activities that give meaning to life and help overcome, or alleviate, the burden of symptoms temporarily. During therapy, elements from the three boxes are combined *from the start through the ending*. An example would be that from toolbox X, e.g., social participation—in any form—is a topic already from the start of therapy and parallels with elements from toolbox R, self-regulation techniques, and toolbox E, trauma work in any form [49]. One example could be having a cup of tea with a sister that was also abused as a child. Different elements from the toolboxes REX are paralleled with support from the app environment.

3.3 Inside the app environment

In our DOCs, we provide personalized, need-driven treatment. Patients connect with their assigned clinician using the app. After connection, they automatically receive instructions on how to operate the app environment, as well as an invitation to already start filling the app with personal information. First, patients fill out their personal profile. The planner facilitates planning and organizing significant events and therapy sessions. The planner also facilitates typing cognitions and experiences before the event is happening. Moreover, it facilitates recording anticipatory emotions for that significant event using swipe techniques for levels of arousal. To enhance success, the option of setting a reminder for this event is given. The planner then shows the events and time during the day and asks if the event, e.g., exposure assignment, was performed. In the case of Yes, one can add text to keep notes of this exposure session, accompanied by recording emotional experiencing, mood, and the option of filling out a cognitive schema. However, in the case of No, when the exposure session was not performed, one is reassured and asked what to do next: perform later today or change/alter session. Even canceling is possible, after which again a reassurance message is given with the invitation to plan something else that day, preferably an X-factor activity to lift one's mood. Next patients start using the tracker for registering mood three times a day and activating the steps tracker. Here, patients can access past event-related information and keep diary for significant events during the week, register mood, registering associated emotional experiencing, and (optionally) the first sections of a cognitive schema. Also, they can access notes given by the therapist associated with therapy sessions. Using the support button, the patient can start a chat session with app support or with the therapist. Also, the patient can initiate a VCP session, with and without visual contact, e.g., to team up with the therapist for an online therapist-assisted exposure assignment.

The therapist using the portal side of the app environment is able to connect with the patient upon invitation and access the patient's information filled out in the app. The therapist can overview all patients and their app content in a dashboard in order to reply to need-driven activity and contact requests. Moreover, graphs are presented per patients with regard to mood, emotional experiences, activities, and results from "homework," e.g., exposure exercises, cognitive elaborations, and social activities. Also, sensor-based information from the smartphone environment, as well as EMA-based information, is presented per patient at the therapist's request. Next therapists are able to initiate VCP, chatting, push messages for encouragement, and planning of next VCP session, activities, and treatment exercises for patients. As part of the treatment via chat messaging, web information is sent on topics of patient's personal relevance, e.g., food, physical exercises, lifestyle, psycho-education on PTSD, and trauma symptoms. Also, vlog or blog information of experiences of trauma therapy of other patients can be shared.

3.4 Treatment

3.4.1 Assessment, self-reported EMA, and predictors of therapy course, effectivity, and erosion

For assessment, the VC option in the app is used for intake purposes, clinical interviewing using MINI 5 for the presence of any mental disorder [50] and CAPS 5 for the presence of PTSD [51], and visual clinical assessment. Initial assessments can help determine possible treatment options using self-report measures, e.g., LEC-5 [52] and post-traumatic stress disorder checklist for DSM-5 (PCL-5 [53]) or the Short PTSD Rating Interview (SPRINT; [54]), or for more complex trauma histories or symptoms, the Structured Interview for DESNOS-revised self-report (SIDES-rev-sr; [47, 55]) is sent. Working alliance is regularly measured with the patient and therapist version of the Working Alliance Inventory (WAI; [56]).

Inhibitory and excitatory forms of self-dysregulation are assessed for:

- Problems in affect regulation involve under-regulation and overregulation of affect [15]. Overregulation of affect is assessed with the Bermond-Vorst Alexithymia Questionnaire (BVAQ; [57]), a Dutch 40-item questionnaire with demonstrated psychometric qualities [57]. Under-regulation is assessed with the "Affect instability scale" from the BPDSI [58]. BPDSI scores range from 0 = never to 10 = daily (Cronbach's alpha = .81).

- Relational impairment and adult relational fears involve "fear of abandonment" and "fear of closeness" (e.g., [25, 26]), which are assessed using the Dutch version of the validated 30-item Relationship Style Questionnaire (RSQ; [59]).

- Dissociation involves positive and negative psychoform and somatoform features [15] and is assessed with the Dissociative Experiences Scale (DES; [60]) for negative (e.g., amnesia) and positive (e.g., intrusions) psychoform features and with the Somatoform Dissociation Questionnaire (SDQ-20; [61]) for negative (e.g., anesthesia, paralysis) and positive (e.g., pain, cramps; [24, 26]) somatoform features.

3.4.2 Evidence-based psychotherapy protocols for trauma-related disorders

Using the videoconferencing psychotherapy (VCP) option, we provide psycho-education about the aftermath of (interpersonal) trauma, PTSD symptoms, and the broader scope of DESNOS/DTD symptoms.

When necessary, psycho-education with regard to dissociation and insecure attachment styles is provided. Since many patients suffering from the aftermath of severe trauma have already tried (and often failed) forms of psychotherapy, motivational interviewing combined with the positive aspects and benefits of our app possibilities is provided.

Evidence-based CBT therapies (many publications, e.g., [62]) like imaginal exposure (IE) aiming at extinction of intrusion symptoms, cognitive therapy (CT) aiming at restructuring trauma-related cognitions and beliefs, and eye movement desensitization and reprocessing (EMDR) protocol using clicks and self-initiated bilateral stimulation aiming at reducing intrusion symptoms and overcoming avoidance, or Imagery Rescripting (ImRs) evidence-based protocols for trauma-related disorders may be provided to patients. Next to these directly trauma-focused therapy forms, interpersonal psychotherapy (IPT; [63]) for PTSD is an option aiming at social and relational rehabilitation while focusing on "role transitions" [63].

Network-oriented interventions are provided with data input from EMA. Self- and affect dysregulation and skill development therapy based on network theory and information from EMA with regard to personalized insecure attachment-based self-regulation symptoms and behaviors will be targeted with EMAI and encompass (i) interventions which "directly change the state of one or more symptoms," (ii) protocols oriented to "inhibition of triggering causes," and (iii) protocols oriented at "inhibiting or modifying symptom-symptom connections." For trauma-related symptoms, aiming at "inhibiting or modifying symptom-symptom connections," the therapeutic environment of our DOCs seems very well suited.

3.4.3 Tracking, app-generated EMA, and predictors of therapy course, effectivity, and erosion

The aim here is building skills to self-regulate [64–67] by monitoring therapy gains and relapse prevention based on EMA data using tracking, self-reports, and clinical observations. Tracking in the app environment taps moment-to-moment tracking of emotions and emotional functioning, mood, movement, behavioral activation and physical exercises, and heart rate information derived from smartphone, combined diary and therapeutic notes, mood before and after events, cognitions and beliefs, cognitive schema, and social network. Also, the planner is used for planning VCP moments, exposure exercises, social events, etc. that can be evaluated with mood charts and cognitive reports before, during, and after the events. Also the therapist can make notes for the patient or send push messages. The built-in sensors synchronizing with Google Fit/Apple Healthkit collect data to reflect physical well-being, activity, and lifestyle. The app facilitates personalized medicine/matched care. Results are combined and discussed in a multidisciplinary team using network theory. Psychotherapy indication is concluded upon, as well as matching a psychotherapist for treatment.

Based on results from assessment, EMA information, predictors (facilitating and disruptive) of therapy course, effectivity, and erosion are drawn. During therapy, these symptoms and behaviors will receive special attention to try to augment treatment effectivity of otherwise evidence-based treatments. Before ending treatment, results will also be integrated in a personalized relapse-prevention plan.

3.4.4 Ending the treatment and the working alliance

Ending of treatment and ending of working alliance—albeit in a 100% online environment—is highly comparable to ending of a regular therapeutic environment. However, next to the VCP session, patients have also developed a relation with the app environment, for some, comparable to the bonding with a personal diary.

Within the app, the integrative and personalized relapse-prevention plan is integrated, accompanied by a "selfideo," a video in which the patient speaks to him/herself in a kind and encouraging manner. The content is an abstract of course of treatment with the treatment rationale, memorabilia (mental representations of personal victories/highlights of therapy and low points of therapy course with lessons learned), names of significant helpful others, and a forecast of whatever the (fearless/depressedless) future may hold for them.

Next, a traffic light principle is held: green for subclinical symptomatology, red for clinical diagnosis (relapse), and orange for trigger points that may predict transfer to relapse. These triggers can be, e.g., reduced sleep quality, feelings of stress for more than 3 days, over- or under-eating, skipping sports and social activities, etc. The target here is to prevent crossing the border from "orange" to "red."

At the end of therapy, our patients with complex trauma histories have overcome hysteresis effect to some extent (e.g., avoidance and intrusion of trauma triggers), report no or less dysfunctional self- and affect regulation, and report a more balanced activity of the FEAR, RAGE, and PANIC/GRIEF systems with SEEKING, CARE, and PLAY systems as can be concluded from the app content (EMA).

Longitudinal outcome studies and studies of outcome predictors are currently in preparation.

4. Conclusion

The life-span sequelae of exposure to interpersonal psychological trauma (emotional or physical neglect or abuse or sexual abuse) in childhood, particularly when a primary caretaker is involved, do not seem to be encompassed by any single DSM disorder and interfere with the development of self-regulation skills and development and remainder of homeostasis. Although symptoms include and extend symptoms associated with PTSD with and without dissociative symptoms, it has been argued that these sequelae also include a complex symptom presentation reflecting disturbances in (interpersonal) self-regulatory capacities and mental disorders that may occur comorbidly with or separately from PTSD. Whether these sequelae are best understood as a complex variant of PTSD (CPTSD), or a complicated array of overlapping mental and personality disorders, is controversial. However, there is mounting evidence that a disorder of extreme stress not otherwise specified (DESNOS) formulation of CPTSD or in childhood, adolescence, and young adulthood (YA), developmental trauma disorder (DTD) constitutes a distinct syndrome of potential clinical utility. Three core features of DESNOS/DTD are affect dysregulation, identity alterations (dissociation), and relational impairment (insecure attachment) and empirically have been associated with qualitatively different and dysfunctional self-regulation vicious cycles: inhibitory, excitatory, and combined inhibitory and excitatory (IE) dysregulation. These can be also considered as trans-diagnostic symptoms clustered along the lines of the network theory.

Individuals with mental health problems may face barriers to accessing effective psychotherapies, e.g., waiting lists in general mental health institutions or office hours [68]. People are becoming more and more supported by technology, and many people use smartphones with apps. Therefore we initiated DOCs using smartphone app for VCP. Our DOCs provide with technology-supported evidence-based treatment in patients' environments and at their convenience in an app environment. Also, it facilitates continuously gathering real-time sensor- and self-reported data that facilitates assessment, self-reported EMA, and need-driven treatment and helps target predictors of therapy course, effectivity, and erosion. Treatment is successful when patients with complex trauma histories have overcome hysteresis effect to some extent (e.g., avoidance and intrusion of trauma triggers), report no or less dysfunctional self- and affect regulation, and report a more balanced activity of the FEAR, RAGE, and PANIC/GRIEF systems with SEEKING, CARE, and PLAY systems as can be concluded from the app content (EMA). Also, they have learned that behavior promotes resilience and prevents relapse. The integrative treatment as described aims to encompass the best of both worlds: it combines established evidence-based treatment protocols for PTSD with innovative technology-enriched app environment that captures more complex trauma-related symptoms and behaviors (lifestyle) to augment therapy effect, improve quality of life, and prevent relapse. However, our work remains a "work in progress": a continuous improvement of technology-supported evidence-based treatment.

Author details

Annemiek van Dijke[1]* and Jacques van Lankveld[2]

1 Parnassia|psyQ and Niceday, Amsterdam, The Netherlands

2 Open University, Heerlen, The Netherlands

*Address all correspondence to: a.vandijke@psyQ.nl

References

[1] Kaffman A. The silent epidemic of neurodevelopmental injuries. Biological Psychiatry. 2009;(7):624-626

[2] van der Kolk BA, Roth S, Pelcovitz D, Sunday S, Spinazzola J. Disorders of extreme stress: The empirical foundation of a complex adaptation to trauma. Journal of Traumatic Stress. 2005;**18**:389-399. DOI: 10.1002/jts.20047

[3] D'Andrea W, Ford JD, Stolbach B, Spinazzola J, van der Kolk BA. Under-standing interpersonal trauma in children: Why we need a developmentally appropriate trauma diagnosis. American Journal of Orthopsychiatry. 2012;**2**:187-200. DOI: 10.1111/j.1939-0025.2012.01154.x

[4] Landy MSH, Wagner AC, Brown-Bowers A, Monson CM. Examining the evidence for complex posttraumatic stress disorder as a clinical diagnosis. Journal of Aggression, Maltreatment & Trauma. 2015;**24**:215-236. DOI: 10.1080/10926771.2015.1002649

[5] Resick PA, Bovin MJ, Calloway AL, Dick AM, King MW, Mitchell KS, et al. A critical evaluation of the complex PTSD literature: Implications for DSM-5. Journal of Traumatic Stress. 2012;**25**:241-251. DOI: 10.1002/jts.21699

[6] Ford JD, Courtois CA. Complex PTSD, affect dysregulation, and borderline personality disorder. Borderline Personality Disorder and Emotion Dysregulation. 2014;**1**:9. DOI: 10.1186/2051-6673-1-9

[7] van Dijke A, Hopman JAB, Ford JD. Affect dysregulation, psychoform dissociation, and adult relational fears mediate the relationship between childhood trauma and complex posttraumatic stress disorder independent of the symptoms of borderline personality disorder. European Journal of Psychotraumatology. 2018;**9**(1):1400878. DOI: 10.1080/20008198.2017.1400878

[8] Ford JD. Complex trauma and complex PTSD. In: Cook J, Gold S, Dalenberg C, editors. Handbook of Trauma Psychology. Washington, DC: American Psychological Association; 2017. pp. 322-349

[9] Ford JD. Complex PTSD: Research directions for nosology/assessment, treatment, and public health. European Journal of Psychotraumatology. 2015;**6**:27584. DOI: 10.3402/ejpt.v6.27584

[10] Knefel M, Garvert DW, Cloitre M, Lueger-Schuster B. Update to an evaluation of ICD-11 PTSD and complex PTSD criteria in a sample of adult survivors of childhood institutional abuse by Knefel & Lueger-Schuster (2013): A latent profile analysis. European Journal of Psychotraumatology. 2015;**6**:25290. DOI: 10.3402/ejpt.v6.25290

[11] Knefel M, Lueger-Schuster B. An evaluation of ICD-11 PTSD and complex PTSD criteria in a sample of adult survivors of childhood institutional abuse. European Journal of Psychotraumatology. 2013;**4**. DOI: 10.3402/ejpt.v4i0.22608

[12] Cloitre M, Garvert DW, Brewin CR, Bryant RA, Maercker A. Evidence for proposed ICD-11 PTSD and complex PTSD: A latent profile analysis. European Journal of Psychotraumatology. 2013;**4**. DOI: 10.3402/ejpt.v4i0.20706

[13] Porges SW. The polyvagal theory: New insights into adaptive reactions of the autonomic nervous system. Cleveland Clinic Journal of Medicine. 2009;**76**:90

[14] Van Dijke A, Ford JD, Frank LE, Van Son M, van der Hart O. Association of childhood trauma-by-primary-caregiver and affect dysregulation with borderline personality disorder symptoms in adulthood. Psychological Trauma: Theory, Research, Practice, and Policy. 2013;**5**:217-224. DOI: 10.1037/a0027256

[15] Van Dijke A, Van der Hart O, Ford JD, Van Son M, Van der Heijden, Bühring M. Affect dysregulation and dissociation in borderline personality disorder and somatoform disorder: Differentiating inhibitory and excitatory experiencing states. Journal of Trauma & Dissociation. 2010;**11**:424-443. DOI: 10.1080/15299732.2010.496140

[16] Moormann PP, Bermond B, Vorst HCM, Bloemendaal A, Teijn S, Rood L. New avenues in alexithymia research: The creation of alexithymia types. In: Denollet J, Nyklicek I, Vingerhoets A, editors. Emotion Regulation: Conceptual and Clinical Issues. New York: Springer; 2008. pp. 27-42

[17] Bermond B, Clayton K, Liberova A, Luminet O, Maruszewski T, Ricci Bitti PE, et al. A cognitive and affective dimension of alexithymia in six languages and seven populations. Cognition & Emotion. 2007;**21**:1125-1136

[18] Moormann PP, Albach F, Bermond B, Van Dijke A, De Jong J, Wineke J, et al. Gender differences in the impact of child sexual abuse on alexithymia, dissociation and self. In: Kalfoglou EA, editor. Sexual Abuse—Breaking the Silence. InTech; 2012. ISBN 979-953-307-685-9

[19] Bermond B, Moormann PP, Albach F. The VDA impact of severe childhood sexual abuse on the development of alexithymia in adulthood. Psychotherapy and Psychosomatics. 2008;**77**:260-262

[20] Lane RD, Weihs KL, Herring A, Hishaw A, Smith R. Affective agnosia: Expansion of the alexithymia construct and a new opportunity to integrate and extend Freud's legacy. Neuroscience and Biobehavor Review. 2015;**55**:594-611

[21] Van Dijke A, Ford JD, Frank LE, van der Hart O. Association of childhood complex trauma and dissociation with complex posttraumatic stress disorder symptoms in adulthood. Journal of Trauma & Dissociation. 2015;**16**:428-441. DOI: 10.1080/15299732.2015.1016253

[22] Ford JD. Dissociation in complex posttraumatic stress disorder or disorders of extreme stress not otherwise specified (DESNOS). In: Dell PF, O'Neill JA, Somer E, editors. Dissociation and The Dissociative Disorders: DSM-V and Beyond. New York: Routledge; 2009. pp. 471-485

[23] Van der Hart O, Nijenhuis ER, Steele K. Dissociation: An insufficiently recognized major feature of complex posttraumatic stress disorder. Journal of Traumatic Stress. 2005;**18**:413-423. DOI: 10.1002/jts.20049

[24] Van der Hart O, Van Dijke A, Van Son M, Steele K. Somatoform dissociation in traumatized World War I Combat Soldiers: A neglected. Clinical Heritage Journal of Trauma and Dissociation. 2000;**1**:33-66

[25] Van Dijke A, Ford JD. Adult attachment fears and emotion dysregulation in borderline personality and somatoform disorders. Borderline Personality Disorder and Emotion Dysregulation. 2015;**2**:6. DOI: 10.1186/s40479-015-0026-9

[26] Roisman GI, Holland A, Fortuna K, Fraley RC, Clausell E, Clarke A. The Adult Attachment Interview and

self-reports of attachment style: An empirical rap-prochement. Journal of Personality and Social Psychology. 2007;**92**:678-697. DOI: 10.1037/0022-3514.92.4.678

[27] Fortuna K, Roisman GI. Insecurity, stress, and symptoms of psychopathology: Contrasting results from self-reports versus interviews of adult attachment. Attachment and Human Development. 2008;**10**:11-28. DOI: 10.1080/14616730701868571

[28] Cloitre M, Garvert DW, Weiss B, Carlson EB, Bryant RA. Distinguishing PTSD, complex PTSD, and borderline personality disorder: A latent class analysis. European Journal of Psychotraumatology. 2014;**5**. DOI: 10.3402/ejpt.v5.25097

[29] Dorahy MJ, Middleton W, Deager K, McGurrin P, Williams M, Chambers R. Dissociation, shame, complex PTSD, child maltreatment and intimate relation-ship self-concept in dissociative disorder, chronic PTSD and mixed psychiatric groups. Journal of Affective Disorders. 2014;**172C**:195-203. DOI: 10.1016/j.jad.2014.10.008

[30] Van Dijke A, Ford J, Van der Hart O, Van Son M, Van der Heijden PGM, Bühring M. Complex posttraumatic stress disorder in patients with borderline personality disorder, somatoform disorder, and comorbid borderline personality and somatoform disorders. Psychological Trauma: Theory, Research Practice, and Policy. 2012;**2**:162-168. DOI: 10.1037/a0025732

[31] Borsboom D. A network theory of mental disorders. World Psychiatry. 2017;**16**:1723-8617. DOI: 10.1002/wps.20375

[32] Panksepp J, Biven M. The Archaeology of Mind: Neuroevolutionary Origins of Human Emotions. New York: W.W. Norton & Company, Inc; 2012

[33] Felitti VJ et al. Relationship of childhood abuse and household dysfunction to many of the leading causes of death in adults. American Journal of Preventive Medicine. 1998;**14**:245-258

[34] Burns EE, Fischer S, Jackson JL, Harding HG. Deficits in emotion regulation mediate the relationship between childhood abuse and later eating disorder symptoms. Child Abuse & Neglect. 2012;**36**:32-39. DOI: 10.1016/j.chiabu.2011.08.005

[35] Benton SA, Heesacker M, Snowden SJ, Lee G. Therapist-assisted, online (TAO) intervention for anxiety in college students: TAO outperformed treatment as usual. Professional Psychology: Research and Practice. 2016;**47**:363-371. DOI: 10.1037/pro0000097

[36] Stubbings DR et al. Comparing in-person to videoconference-based cognitive behavioral therapy for mood and anxiety disorders: Randomized controlled trial. Journal of Medical Internet Research. 2013;**15**:11 e258. DOI: 10.2196/jmir.2564

[37] Andrews G, Cuijpers P, Craske MG, McEvoy P, Titov N. Computer therapy for the anxiety and depressive disorders is effective, acceptable and practical health care: A meta-analysis. PLoS One. 2010;**5**:e13196. DOI: 10.1371/journal.pone.0013196

[38] Bouton ME, Todd TP. A fundamental role for context in instrumental learning and extinction. Behavioural Processes. 2014;**104**:13-19. DOI: 10.1016/j.beproc.2014.02.012

[39] Cuijpers P, Donker T, van Straten A, Li J, Andersson G. Is guided self-help as effective as face-to-face psychotherapy for depression and anxiety disorders? A systematic review and meta-analysis of comparative outcome studies. Psychological

Medicine. 2010;**40**:1943-1957. DOI: 0033291710000772

[40] Effting M, Kindt M. Contextual control of human fear associations in a renewal paradigm. Behaviour Research and Therapy. 2007;**45**:2002-2018. DOI: 10.1016/j.brat.2007.02.011

[41] Scholten WD, Batelaan NM, van Balkom AJLM, Penninx BWJH, Smit JH, van Oppen P. Recurrence of anxiety disorders and its predictors. Journal of Affective Disorders. 2013;**147**:180-185. DOI: 10.1016/j.jad.2012.10.031

[42] Bouton ME. A learning theory perspective on lapse, relapse, and the maintenance of behavior change. Health Psychology. 2000;**19**:57-63. DOI: 10.1037/0278-6133.19.Suppl1.57

[43] Bouton ME. Context, ambiguity, and unlearning: Sources of relapse after behavioral extinction. Biological Psychiatry. 2002;**52**:976-986. DOI: 10.1016/S0006-3223(02)01546-9

[44] Simpson SG, Reid C. Therapeutic alliance in videoconferencing psychotherapy: A review. Australian Journal of Rural Health. 2014;**22**:280-299

[45] Ringel S, Faye Mishna F, Sanders J. Developing a reflective self in cyber space. Psychoanalytic Psychology. 2017;(1):87-95

[46] Lewis F, Groves K, Roberts V, Bisson JI. Internet-based guided self-help for posttraumatic stress disorder (PTSD): Randomized controlled trial. Depression and Anxiety. 2017;**34**:555-565. DOI: 10.1002/da.22645

[47] Ford JD, Kidd P. Early childhood trauma and disorders of extreme stress as pre-dictors of treatment outcome with chronic posttraumatic stress disorder. Journal of Traumatic Stress. 1998;**11**:743-761. DOI: 10.1023/A:1024497400891

[48] van der Hart O, Nijenhuis ERS, Steele K. The Haunted Self: Structural Dissociation and the Treatment of Chronic Traumatization. New York: W. W. Norton; 2006

[49] Van Dijke A. The clinical assessment of attachment trauma related self- and affect dysregulation. In: Vingerhoets A, Nyklicek I, Denollet J, editors. Affect Regulation: Conceptual and Clinical Issues. New York: Springer; 2008. pp. 150-169

[50] van Vliet IM, Leroy H, van Megen HJGM. MINI International Neuropsychiatric Interview (M.I.N.I.). Nederlandse versie 5.0.0. 2000

[51] Weathers FW, Blake DD, Schnurr PP, Kaloupek DG, Marx BP, Keane TM. The Clinician-Administered PTSD Scale for DSM-5 (CAPS-5). 2013. Interview available from the National Center for PTSD at www.ptsd.va.gov

[52] Weathers L, Keane P, Marx S. Life Events Checklist for the DSM-5 (LEC 5). National Center for PTSD. 2013. Available from the National Center for PTSD at www.ptsd.va.gov

[53] Blevins CA, Weathers FW, Davis MT, Witte TK, Domino JL. The Posttraumatic Stress Disorder Checklist for DSM-5 (PCL-5): Development and initial psychometric evaluation. Journal of Traumatic Stress. 2015;**28**:489-498

[54] Connor K, Davidson J. SPRINT: A brief global assessment of post-traumatic stress disorder. International Clinical Psychopharmacology. 2001;**16**:279-284

[55] Ford JD, Van Dijke A, Van der Hart O. Self-report version of the Structured Interview for Disorders of Extreme Stress (SIDES-r-nl). Utrecht: Utrecht University; 2002. Unpublished manual

[56] Horvath AO, Greenberg LS. Development and validation of the

Working Alliance Inventory (WAI). Journal of Counseling Psychology. 1989;**36**:223-233

[57] Vorst HCM, Bermond B. Validity and reliability of the Bermond-Vorst Alexithymia Questionnaire. Personality and Individividual Differences. 2001;**30**:413-434

[58] Arntz A, Van den Hoorn M, Cornelis J, Verheul R, Van den Bosch W, De Bie AJHT. Reliability and validity of the borderline personality severity index. Journal of Personality Disorders. 2003;**17**:45-59. DOI: 10.1521/pedi.17.1.45.24053

[59] Griffin D, Batholomew K. Models of the self and other: Fundamental dimensions underlying measures of adult attachment (RSQ). Journal of Personality and Social Psychology. 1994;**67**:430-445. DOI: 10.1037/0022-3514.67.3.430

[60] Bernstein EM, Putnam FW. Development, reliability, and validity of a dissociation scale (DES). Journal of Nervous and Mental Disease. 1986;**174**:727-735. DOI: 10.1097/00005053-198612000-00004

[61] Nijenhuis ERS, Spinhoven P, Van Dyck R, Van der Hart O, Van der Linden J. The development and psychometric characteristics of the Somatoform Dissociation Questionnaire (SDQ-20). Journal of Nervous and Mental Disease. 1996;**184**:688-694. DOI: 10.1097/00005053-199611000-00006

[62] Jung SR. A randomized controlled trial on cognitive restructuring and imagery modification to reduce the feeling of being contaminated in adult survivors of childhood sexual abuse suffering from posttraumatic stress disorder. Psychotherapy and Psychosomatics. 2013;**82**:213-220

[63] Markowitz J. Interpersonal Psychotherapy for Post-traumatic Stress Disorder. Oxford Press; 2017

[64] van Dijke A, Lenstra S, Wineke J, Ford JD. Cognitive-emotional functioning in somatic symptom and related disorders: Self-reports versus observer-rated findings. Journal of Psychology and Psychotherapy. 2016;**6**:271. DOI: 10.4172/2161- 0487.1000271

[65] Bohn D, Bernardy K, Wolfe F, Hauser W. The association among childhood maltreatment, somatic symptom intensity, depression, and somatoform dissociative symptoms in patients with fibromyalgia syndrome: A single-center cohort study. Journal of Trauma and Dissociation. 2013;**14**:342-358. DOI: 10.1080/15299732.2012.736930

[66] Ford JD. Emotion regulation and skills-based interventions. In: Cook J, Gold S, Dalenberg C, editors. Handbook of Trauma Psychology. Vol. 2. Washington, DC: American Psychological Association; 2017. pp. 227-252

[67] Ford JD, Courtois CA, Steele K, Hart O, Nijenhuis ER. Treatment of complex posttraumatic self-dysregulation. Journal of Traumatic Stress. 2005;**18**:437-447. DOI: 10.1002/jts.20051

[68] Kazdin AE, Blase SL. Rebooting psychotherapy research and practice to reduce the burden of mental illness. Perspectives on Psychological Science. 2011;**6**:21-37. DOI: 10.1177/1745691610393527